DON'T EVER

GIVE UP

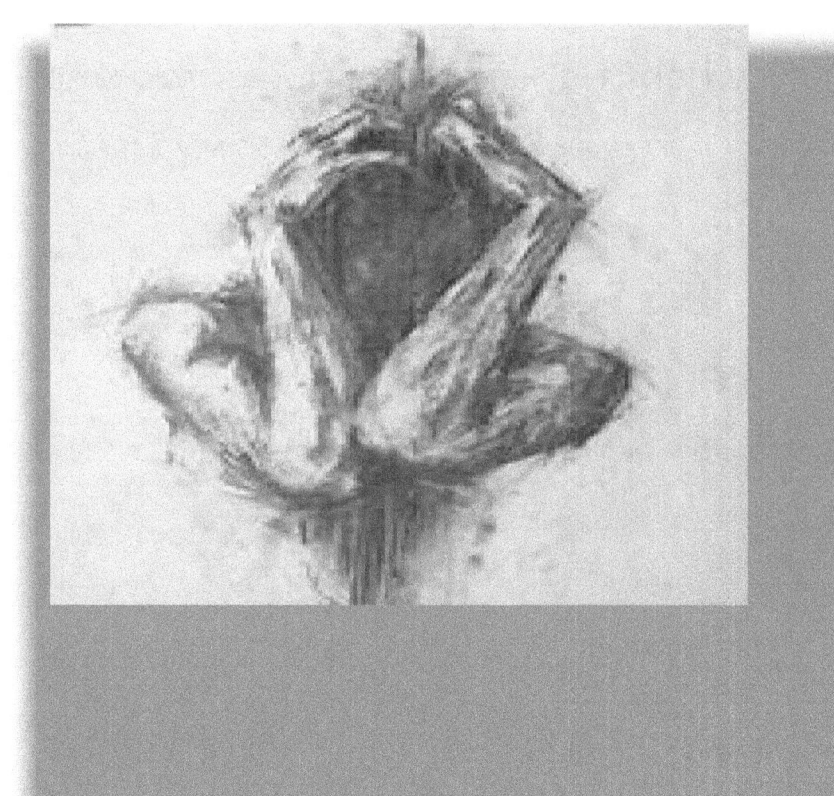

COPING WITH DEPRESSION

A CHRISTIAN PERSPECTIVE

ROBERT C. TAYLOR

DEDICATED TO ONLY TRUE LOVE OF MY LIFE

LORIANN YOU GAVE ME COMFORT

WHEN THE MENTAL PAIN WAS TOO MUCH

THANK YOU FOR SAVING MY LIFE

Twisting its web of fear and great pain

The pain does hide, its welcome far overstayed

Nagging fear tramples all good as it appears

Circular thoughts have captured your mind.

Where do I go how to escape, I know not

Strength arises through faiths strong voice

Very soon, Courage its reigns doth come

Divine truth I hear, and its call I feel

Mortal thoughts will never conquer

Gods Victory cometh and his peace is near

Rest assured, Fathers peace doeth come

It is part of the plan

The burden of mental pain and worry you've carried so long

Your kind savior will carry it all for you, and soon

Why do I fear, doubt and disbelief was mine

Why do I worry, want, or lack faith

Father's Steed of wisdom, is ready to ride

Take wing, fly away from fear and pain

Salvation reigns and liberty, it is soon yours

Faith is your ride and fears is your captor

Faith's abundance doeth crush fears head

Pure is his atonement and real it doeth heal

Come forth my son, fear not and only believe

A new day is yours, breath and live again

A perfect brightness of hope does shine forth

The love and peace of the Savior you do have

Miracles are of God they soon will be yours

Step forward out of the dark my son and light it doeth shine

Your loneliness is no more, the fathers love it doeth replace

The Father, The Son their infinite love is with you evermore.

2

CLINICAL VS PSYCHOLOGICAL DEPRESSION

CLINICAL DEPRESSION is an invisible silent physiological disease causing a chemical change in your brain that leads to an emotional disorder. People feel compassion toward those individuals suffering from cancer because they can see the outward affects cancer has on them. A majority of individuals that you interact with you can't feel compassion for the suffering you feel from Clinical Depression because they don't believe in what they can't see.

PSYCHOLOGICAL DEPRESSION is not a disease. It is brought on usually by a difficult event in life such as the death of a loved one, a divorce, a severe break up of a relationship and many other difficult things that life brings.

The main difference between the Clinical and Psychological Depression is the intensity of the mental and physical symptoms. Clinical Depression is accompanied by relentless mental. You can work out, you can do activities that you enjoy, you can eat one of your favorite foods and the pain from Clinical Depression will still be there. You can do certain things that will alleviate the mental symptoms of Psychological Depression away such as working out or eating one of your favorite foods. You will often hear this comment " I feel much better after working out" or they will go get a chocolate milkshake and comment " Well that really helped that hit the spot". With Clinical Depression doing those specific things will not take the pain away.

3

<u>THE UGLY TRUTH ABOUT DEPRESSION</u>

Depression is a lifelong battle that is not a respecter of people, places, or events. Depression is so devastating because it affects the brain and the brain is the engine for your life. Your thoughts are 100% consumed and replaced with the mental pain from Depression which makes it a constant struggle to be able to focus on the things at hand.

The best way to describe Depression is if there was a magic wand across the room that would heal Depression instantly it would be too big of a hassle to go over and get the wand.

Depression freezes you, it is immobilizing, and you literally feel paralyzed. With Depression, you live in a pseudo or false reality and you live in a reality that is completely different than others. While not a thought is given by most individuals about being able to just walk normally down the street, this is a difficult task for those suffering from Depression, because you have such harsh pain, it is hard to walk, to carry on a conversation, to focus on your work, and to emotionally connect with other individuals, When you suffer You perceive the world very differently than a normal person, and you feel that people are constantly looking at you and judging you.

There are several different segments of Mental Illness, Schizophrenia, Psychosis, Anxiety, Eating Disorders and Social Phobias. On a regular basis, the news will have stories of crimes and murders that are linked to Mental Illness such as the Unabomber who suffered from Social Disorder and Psychosis and the lady who drowned her 5 children who suffered from Schizophrenia. The list of crimes committed by individual's sufferings from Depression is almost nonexistent. Depression is not schizophrenia or psychosis and the only harm that individuals do when they are having Depression is to commit suicide. The press has mislabeled Mental Illness incorrectly and it is often times lumped with Schizophrenia

The late great Winston Churchill suffered from Depression, as did Mike Wallace of 60 Minutes and Michael Phelps possibly the greatest athlete ever suffers from Depression.

Early on while suffering from the disease, I viewed people with Depression as weak individuals, therefore, and I was unwilling to accept that I may be suffering from Depression. If I would have accepted that I had Depression sooner, I would have recovered 10 Yrs sooner.

Society doesn't talk openly about Depression because the majority of individuals view you as weak if you have Depression. If you tell a prospective employer about your Depression your chances of getting the job will be decreased, you will be treated differently if people know you have Depression, you could be ostracized by certain individuals, your friends could alienate you and some people will just view you as weird and different. It is all very unfair, but until the Depression is fully understood by the public it will always be that way.

Depression is the most depraved disease that a person can have and is the hardest trials that an individual can face. If you have diabetes, you can use your brain to deal with the disease, but when you have Depression it is your brain that is affected so the very tool that you use to deal with your disease has the disease itself. It affects your thoughts every single second of the day and you feel the emotional pain with every effort, movement, thought, word, and action you take during the day. The pain at times can be literally excruciating, insatiable in its nature and relentless. If you are going to make it through this trial and succeed in overcoming this disease you are going to have to be very tough, and you can in no way be weak. The weak with this disease are those men that end up killing themselves. I can promise you that if you don't take a stand against this disease that you will end up committing suicide. In my opinion, this is absolutely the hard disease on the planet to deal with. This is the mother of all diseases to have, it sucks so badly, and the emotional pain associated with this disease has no limit to how bad you can feel and as too how long you will feel the pain. So, buckle up and prepare yourself for the hardest trial that you will face your entire life

---

DO YOU HAVE DEPRESSION

I first got sick on December 18th, 1983 at 7:35. It started with dizziness and disorientation. I had no idea what was wrong and thought that I would wake up the next day and feel fine. I woke up the next morning only to feel even worse with a severe headache and incredible mental fog. Every day I woke up with several different symptoms including the following

- Insatiable relentless mental pain

- Severe Headaches

- Mental Fogginess

- Severe Nausea

- Disoriented

- Head felt like it was asleep

- Extreme Dizziness

- Arms went to sleep

- Legs went to sleep

- Incredible muscle tightness through my entire body

- Severe Chest Pains

- Severe Anxiety

- Severe feeling of fear

- Severe feeling that I was going to fall off the face of the earth at any moment.

- People avoidance being around people caused me physical and emotional pain

- Panic Attacks

- Shortness of Breath

- Inability to concentration

- Inability to talk clearly

- Inability to remember words or names

So, what I recommend at this point, is you go to your Family Physician and have him do a complete physical including as many blood panel workups as possible. If you can afford it, I would suggest that you have an MRI and EKG also.

You will find that all your results will come back normal and you will be declared in good health. You will be wishing in your mind that there is something wrong with you because you won't be able to comprehend that you can have so many physical and symptoms and there not be anything wrong with you. It will not make any sense to you that you are fine. When you are declared in good physical health and you still feel physically and emotionally terrible you most likely have Depression.

I will tell you a little bit about my journey so that you will not be prone to make the same mistakes that I made. When I first got Depression, I suffered with it for a few years, but finally decided to have a comprehensive medical analysis done. So, I flew to Calgary Canada in the middle of winter from Newport Beach to meet my parents to have several specialists complete an exhaustive physical workup on me. When we flew into Calgary it was 45 degrees below zero. My wife Loriann only had on short shoes and no socks yet we had to walk 3 blocks to our Hotel, and it was so cold. The Doctors ran every physical test there was and completed all the necessary blood test. Guess what, I was 100% percent fine.

The only thing that came about as a result of our trip to Canada, is my Dad's partner put me on Xanax, a nightmare drug that led to Hallucinations and all sorts of problems for me. DON'T LET A GENERAL PRACTITIONER PUT YOU ON ANY OLD DRUG.

So, one of the major problems that I had was insatiable nausea. I went to at least 5 different doctors spending hundreds of dollars and guess what, nothing was wrong with my stomach and it was a complete waste of time. SO BE AWARE THAT NAUSEA IS A VERY TYPICAL SYMPTOM

So, I took a very drastic kind of embarrassing tactic. I decided to go to Hospital Santa Monica located in Ensenada Mexico. I stayed there for 6 weeks on a comprehensive approach where they did Hydrogen Peroxide Intravenous drips daily. To say the least, it did nothing for me, except make me feel complete embarrassment for going there. One minor thing did occur is that was positive. I met their therapist in training, and we would meet and talk 3 times per week, helping me to realize that Talk Therapy does help, but it did not cure my physical and emotional symptoms. TALK THERAPY IS ONLY ONE OF THE PIECES OF THE PUZZLE, IT IS NOT THE CURE.

So being desperately sick, my wife and I were willing to do almost anything to get me feeling better. My wife suggested that I quit my job for a bit until I feel better. I started to fly to Utah once a week to see a lady that did a very aggressive upper body massage using her elbow on my back and on my stomach and after that treatment, I would go over and have a Colonic. I was able to rid myself of my severe headaches and my nausea with these treatments. The first relief of my physical symptoms from Depression and it felt so good to be rid of my nausea. To this day I still employ the massage techniques on my stomach and I still do at least 2 enemas per week to keep my nausea at bay.

5

<u>HEAVENLY FATHER IS ON YOUR SIDE</u>

I am so appreciative to be able to feel deeply, I think it is one of the greatest approbations of the spirit that God will give to us, the ability to feel deeply. When you feel deeply you are advantaged to have access to those painfully sweet Godly feelings. You cry more, you see people for who they really are, children of God, you see circumstances from a position of love and not judgment.

It hasn't always been that way for myself, I have had to come to ascertain that when I feel mental pain from Depression, that I am literally being schooled and refined. I used to feel great trepidation of the thought of being refined and facing my mental pain, I looked at it like a nuisance or its just dumb pain, oh, how far from the reality of life was I. I am so grateful for the pain of adversity and trials and for having to face this mental pain, the inexplicable thing is that if you submit to god with your pain, then a stark, soft, sweetness comes from the harsh reality of your circumstances. Being born again and ridding myself of the natural man were once again words on a page, it was a goal, a thing that I wanted to be able to do, but I didn't feel it. Well, those words are real, and the power to change is real.

The only way to know this is thru experience and going down a road and coming to a fork and choosing one of the two paths being bitter or submission to Go, I took the bitter path and failed, and thru experience went down the Submission to God path. To open the gate to the Submission to God path you will need the key to the gate which is Humility and that key can be very difficult to find and at times it may seem like you will never find it.

Saying audibly to god on your knees in your room with tears sullying your comforter; O Father, I submit myself to you and this mental pain, let my will be swallowed up in thine, please show me the way and let this mental pain distill me, let me have the pure love of Christ in my heart, help me to have no guile, help me to forgive one and all, succor me to be slow to anger, help me to love everyone, help me not to judge, but to give the benefit of the doubt to all men and women.

This does not happen by kneeling once, or twice or even kneeling several times, it happens when your eyes smolder and sting over and over because of the unadorned substance of your tears. It really is only one thing and one thing only it's a miracle. God can amend your heart and he is the only one who can do it. Yes your plight in life may take a wrong course, and you may judge others, and may at times be quick to anger, and your tongue may cut like a sword, but when you kneel with father, who is there no matter what happens in your life and say, Father please let me feel this prayer and let me really sincerely talk to you now about how much I am hurting, he will attend you and you will feel that simple spirit in your heart, the familiar tears will come forward and guess what, Heavenly Father listens and I really don't know how it happens, what physiological, spiritual or emotional changes that take place, but at that moment you are a changed person, the power of God has indelibly touched your life.

 Now you may transgress, you may make some sobering errors, but the simplest truth of God's reality is that when you retire to that place of comfort next to your bed, father is convening right next to you, and it's if he softly touches your shoulder, letting you know that he's there and he whispers quietly, we can make it together through this pain today, tomorrow, and always.

The most profound detail about it is that you really change as a creature, you don't get a better job, you don't drive a better car, your problems do not dissipate or vanish, but you see his children for who they are, you perceive other's needs, you feel their pain, your desire to love others becomes insatiable and others start to become the nucleus of your thoughts. It isn't about you any longer and your pain, it's about loving others. Love is the true power of God and love really does disentangle all problems. The strenuous part is getting enough humility and taking the actions such that you let Heavenly Father heal your heart and your heart starts to heal others.

I trust in these principles, but only speak as an applicant, a participant, not as a teacher, I am far removed from leading saints down the footpath of love. I gaze back at my life and in my heart, I find it hard to consider that I was ever mean in the past, I can't really feel meanness anymore, I find it hard that I have ever fostered anger or elevated my voice to my loved ones. I am not good at these things, but I can tell you that I feel these things deeply.

I know too that I can withdraw to that secure habitation in my chambers and figure out how to do things better with Heavenly Father. Does the pain halt, no it doesn't, sometimes it gets crueler, and sometimes it gets so depraved that I can't impede the tears from emanating, but I do grasp, and I testify that Heavenly Father's existence is true, his love is real and unfeigned and that the most heartwarming thing that I have been subjected to is, being able to allow the power of God to amend my person?

My testimony is so much stouter and my belief in Heavenly Father 's love and Jesus's Christ teachings are felt even more deeply and intensely than in years past, and why, because I made a natural decision because of my pain to submit to God.

Being able to feel love for people more fully, comes from the arduous task of submitting myself to the will of God, once again I am a student, not a teacher and do not confess supremacy over these principles. I am about feeling the soft, serene, and peaceable feelings that Heavenly Father can bequeath to us if we will only submit.

Oh, have I been lonely, so very lonely there were instances that I believed I wouldn't be able to arise from the floor, but I did arise, and I moved forward with faith. If you will only refuse to not listen to the constant siren of thought "don't believe don't have faith, but instead submit and pray to Heavenly Father, please let my heart be filled with the pure love of Christ

My parents unwearyingly taught me the principles of the gospel, and I feel gratitude every single day for what they taught me. Sometimes during my loneliest travails, I have felt my mom and dad' spirits, not in a peculiar way, but I can feel their tears for me, and I feel the deep love they still have for me across the veil, they are my silent cheering section.

In my life I have tried to do right, I loved my mission more than any other thing I have ever done, I married worthily in the temple, I resolved to consecrate my days to our 5 youngsters and to my sweetheart, and that was the solitary fixation I had. All I fancied was there love and respect. I spent an inordinate time with my children and together we taught them correct principles and enjoyed raising our babies. I held my wife in high esteem and resolved to do all I knew within my power and knowledge at that time, to love her and be a faithful partner.

I have battled clinical depression for over 30 years. Instead of acting out maliciously because of the illness, I would just say to my sweetheart, I don't feel good, could I possibly bury my tears in your neck, she would give me that little look of love that would melt me and she always obliged, and was unceasingly empathetic to me.

Sometimes free agency can seem like the most depraved thing that we have in the gospel, and at the time, the consequences of free agency are piercingly hard in their effect. Well, the love of my life broke my heart, and freely acted on her free agency to adjourn the earthly partnership we had. Granting my imperfections, I have at times, said things I shouldn't, but love may fleet away at times, but the love you felt for someone is always there. I still love her today as much as the day she left and am continually pulled back to my family, by the unceasing love I feel towards them.

My purpose in life was vacated, the center of my life seemed it had collapsed, and it went away, so very fast, and the feelings attached to that experience were almost too much for me to shoulder. Then when you feel you are going to crumble under the guise of this eternal plan of salvation, you turn to Father, and supplicate him to refine you and fill you full of love, as you persist in your tears at night, you take in what you need from these experiences and you become fascinatingly grateful for the peace he always gives you.

All I wanted was to grow old with my love, but behind others, the free agency which can at times seem ill-informed to you, there are the soft sublime tender mercies of the lord you will softly experience if you will only submit to that free agency, which is oh so hard. God is never mistaken, but we as his children turn the right answer into a mistake because of life's travails. I have suffered emotional and physical challenges, and the pain behind those has seemed to be so colossal at times, and the irony is the sweetness that resides by enduring those colossal experiences is indeed a beautiful mystery to me.

Countless people are sad, brokenhearted, and unhappy. I feel great sorrow for their anguish, some are angry, some are so lonely, some are ready to give up, some have fortunately discovered the joy of submitting to god and there are some that are just absent, are falling out of love, some who don't feel like themselves, others have gone astray and are just of course. It is ok to be all those things. , I am still enduring my trials, inconveniences, and tribulations, but I know the power of submission to father's will and the tangible power of God and love.

There will be brighter days. Although tears, they come in the darkness, there will be light at daybreak. The love of Heavenly Father is exacting in its process, and it has the power to transform you into a creature that loves and feels all things so deeply.

The gospel of Jesus Christ has the preciseness and exactness of how we are to live our lives to return to Father. Jesus Christ's Atonement has the power to transform lives and it does and will.

I have been bruised, tattered, and seemly at times abandoned by life's trials, and this church and gospel are so good. In trials when the fog starts to lift from your mind, and you sense a tiny sliver of clarity, a voice faintly starts to whispers to you, please pray my son, and then you beseech father, and he whispers, again and again, to come to him, you start to have those streams of unceasingly serene tears you've waited for, those tears that have a beautiful peace behind them, you start to trust Father and then the dawn breaks, your humility has paid off and you say, O Father, please, please help me to make sense of this pain, and to have the pure love of Christ in my heart. You start to consider going down the right path, you hesitantly approach the path, which is indeed winding, unstable and wavering, the Heavenly father gives you the unconditional love to traverse the path successfully and you finally know and feel the pure love of Christ inside of you and its undeniable warmth.

6

MAYBE YOU CAN RELATE

SO SCARED

My Depression came on to me instantaneous on December 18th, 1984 at

7:35 pm. I thought that I was getting sick, but with each day I got more

scared. In fact, I felt complete and utter trepidation, I just couldn't believe

that my symptoms were getting worse by the day, the week and by the

month. I have never felt so scared about what was going on in my mind and

body. I didn't feel that I could tell people about what I was experiencing

because I couldn't really define or explain to someone what it. The thing

that was the most frightening was that I thought that it would go away

after I woke up the next day, and I kept that hope alive almost every day

for months until I realized that it wasn't going to go away and that I wasn't

getting any better. Just the thought that every morning I woke up and it

had still there scared me beyond any fear I have ever felt in my life.

NOBODY UNDERSTANDS WHAT ITS LIKE

I was so disappointed how people acted when I told them about what I was

going through. I was so sad to see how my father treated me when I told

him about what I was going through. He told me that I needed to be stronger and that I needed to not think about what I was going through so much. How can you not think about what you are going through when it is part of your mind and body 24 hours a day. I remember telling my best friend about what I was going through and when I was done explaining it, he showed literally zero compassion and acted as if he didn't even understand what I was saying. He quickly changed the topic and acted as if we didn't even talk about it. That was very painful

GOING TO UNIVERSITY WHILE SICK

After I got married, we moved down to Southern California so I could attend the University of Southern California. I was getting two degrees, one in Real Estate Finance and one in Business Entrepreneur. I was so sick when I attended U.S.C. and was in a continual state of dizziness, disorientation and mental fog. My head felt like it was asleep most of the time. I used to have to go to Class 15 minutes early so the dizziness and disorientation would dissipate so that I could focus on the lecture. I remember walking down the sidewalk and have this specific thought. " What would it be like to just walk down the sidewalk and not have to be continually worrying about being dizzy and disoriented?

ZERO HOPE

I reached an emotionally painful mental state I call zero hope as a result of my physical and emotional ailments. There isn't much lower you can go that this state and it means that you have hit bottom emotionally. It takes an awful lot of negative and harsh experiences to be able to arrive at this point.

Absolutely one of the worse things if not the absolute worst thing that I experienced with having Depression is having Zero Hope. There is no place on this universe mentally like when you have Zero Hope. Having Zero Hope is the scariest, most discouraging, disparaging, disheartening, tearful mental states you can ever reach.

I remember I laid on the bed and Loriann just held me in her arms as we both wept for the longest time. Things were not getting better, they were getting worse and we had no idea what was wrong with me and it was just Loriann and me trying to walk this pathway of darkness into nowhere. How do I describe Zero Hope? It just feels like nothingness, there is nothing to see in front of you, you see no future at all, and you are literally stuck in the pain of that moment.

Although it was a horrible position to be in, I do this day feel incredible gratitude to Loriann for holding me in her arms and her never-ending empathy she showed me. It was an awful place to be in but remembering the warmth of her touch and the beauty of her face at that moment is a vivid and beautiful memory for me. I love her so much for the unconditional love compassion and sympathy that she showed me.

Heavenly Father does not let you stay at Zero Hope for very long. I had this growing thought in my mind that I needed to let the universe know that I was not going to have Zero Hope any longer. I have no idea where that thought came from and why I had it. The next day after we lay weeping on the bed, I had this experience. I was walking outside our Apartment Complex called Park Newport which was situated on a beautiful Bluff overlooking back bay in Newport Beach. I was walking along a beautiful walkway and I had a sudden urgent desire to let Heavenly Father and the Universe that I was going to get better. So that is when I literally stated aloud mildly at first and then with fervor then next few time " I am going to get better, I am going to defeat this illness". I really don't understand what happened after I said that, but I never experienced Zero Hope gain and things slowly started to make better sense and we started to learn how to make our way down this path. Zero Hope is from the opposing force Satan who wants us to not have hope because if we don't have hope, then we can't have faith and he has won. Depression will either take you down the path of building your hope and faith or take you down the pathway of despair, it is your choice.

You will ask this question so many times "why is this happening to me" " I am living the gospel and the commandments why is this happening", "what did I do wrong that this is happening to me" "all my dreams are disappearing as result of this" " I'll never get better" " I feel so alone and nobody cares about me". I could go on forever with different questions that you will ask Heavenly Father about why this is happening to you. I sincerely felt that I had been wronged for having to go through this terrible trial.

It is my hope to help you to see down the road and to form the correct perspective of what you are going through in relationship to Heavenly Father wants you to see and how he wants you to proceed. It may be very hard for you to hear these words the way that you are feeling right now, but I wish that I would have known 35 years ago what I know now and could have applied these perspectives that I am discussing.

A true disciples of Christ submit to all trials and you don't get to negotiate with Heavenly Father what trials you will submit to and what trials you won't submit to you. Now currently at this time being a disciple of Christ may not be your priority, so let's put this in a simpler understandable format.

The plan of salvation is a very difficult plan to live. Basically, the plan of Salvation is that when we have any trial and we are feeling bitter about the trial we will go backward and have no progression in our character. Now the interesting part about Heavenly Father powers and how the Atonement of Jesus Christ works is that if we submit to our trials and we get on our knees and tell Heavenly Father that we submit to these trial and that you are willing to drink the bitter cup for as long as Heavenly Father wants you to he will refine you and fill you with pure love Christ. Your trials will excavate your soul and you will not only have a greater spiritual, physical, and mental capacity, but your ability to love others will expand. The greatest thing is that I can promise you're and testify to you from my own personal experiences that you will be able to handle your Depression more effectively and sooner. In other words, it is the highest and the best pathway to take when it comes to this journey that you are on. These words are true, and these are the words that will hopefully make you act and take higher path Heavenly Fathers wants you to take and not to choose the bitter path. The holy ghost is testifying to me as I write this that it is true. I don't know you, but I feel your pain, your aloneness, your fear, your lack of faith, I am with you in spirit, and you can conquer this dreadful disease, please press forward in with increased hope leading to bountiful faith.

PEOPLE HURT ME

Depression causes you to hurt physically and emotionally when you are around people which sounds ludicrous, but it really hurts to be around people, and I don't not the reason to this day. I remember going to Church and literally being scared to be alone with other people around. I always had Loriann at my side. I call it people avoidance, which is a real thing with Depression. To this day I am again grateful to Loriann for not making fun of me or telling me to know when I asked her to be at my side. I now just feel deep gratitude to have had her by my side during those times where it hurt to be around people.

One of the worse places for me to go was into the mall or stores. It was emotionally excruciating to go into those places. It makes you feel weak as a person, it is hard on your self-confidence because you really don't understand why you are feeling that way. If it no longer hurts, you to be around people then you know that you are making progress with your Depression. My Loriann could have brushed me off and but mean, but she never was, she was just so compassionate and empathetic always putting my feelings first before hers.

I was coming home a six-week stay at Hospital Santa Monica in Ensenada. I was driving home, and her family was at our apartment. I was so afraid of seeing her family, so I asked her if she would meet me at the Clubhouse of our apartment building and we could enter the apartment to see her family together. She happily agreed and held my hand and we met her family. That sounds so weak and lame and like I am a pathetic human being, but it is real. Love fills my heart for Loriann for lovingly guiding me through that incredible feeble, weak, and humbly submissive time.

I AM SO TIRED ALL THE TIME

It is unbelievable how tired you are when you suffer from this disease. You are always tired and looking for the next opportunity to sleep. I remember when Loriann said that I needed to stop working for a while and just take some time off. We had just had our first child Bridget, so I stayed at home with Bridget while Loriann taught school. It was so kind of Loriann to have me quit working and have her take over earning the income for the family, so unselfish, but it was very hard for me to take of Bridget because all I wanted to do was sleep. A brand-new baby and a toddler don't want a father that only wants to sleep. I would put her to sleep for a nap and I felt so relieved that I could go back to sleep, but the problem is that her soother or what we call her Binkie would fall out of her mouth and she would wake up and cry. Her blanket would also come unraveled which also would wake her up. So as a clinically depressed person would do, I taped her binky to her mouth with electrician tape. I also got duct tape and wrapped her blanket with it, so she was all cozy. I know some of you will think what a pathetic father, but I was just so tired I would do almost anything to be able to sleep. One thing that I was religious about despite my illness, was trying to stay in decent physical shape.

There was a very beautiful road that went along the back bay by our apartment complex. Every day about 4 pm I would attempt to run around the 4-mile loop of back bay. Most of the days I could hardly put one foot in front of another because I was just so completely exhausted, but I must tell you that I continued running every day for 4 years and towards the end, I did finally reach my goal of running 12 miles straight.

I remember I was running to the music of the Los Angeles Olympics " One Moment in Time " by Whitney Houston. I had persevered over those 4 years and no matter how tired I was I went every day. Finally, I was able to run around the loop 4 times for a total of 12 miles. As I was approaching the end of my run and "One Moment in Time " was playing, I literally stopped and broke down in tears, I had persevered and had a small victory over my Depression. I sat by the side of the roadside and cried with victorious tears because I had defeated the tiredness. It felt a little pathetic that my victory in my life at that time was being able to run 12 miles and overcome a part of my illness and the tiredness, while others were out gainfully started companies, had great jobs and others where developing new and productive relationships with others. But that was my victory and to this day I look at it as a victory and I am proud of it, although small and maybe kind of dumb to some people it was very real for me. And of course, Loriann was just as happy for me.

I HATE HAPPY PEOPLE

One of the most painful things you will experience with Depression is you just don't feel good and you don't feel happy. When you have Depression, you feel grumpy interacting with other individuals. I was washing my car at Newport Beach Self Service Car wash and there was a couple of people that were having the greatest time washing their car together, they were smiling, playful, talkative, and fully enjoying the experience. I remember thinking to myself " I hate how happy you are" " I wish you both would just shut up" " I can't stand you both" Isn't that a terrible way to feel, but it is a thing that happens with this insidious disease. It just can't be helped it is how you really feel. All I can say is get through it

IM SO AGGRESSIVE

Depression puts you in a bad mood and it also causes some of your worse characteristics to come out at the worse times. So, you must be cognizant of your weaknesses and make sure that Depression doesn't emphasize those bad characteristics. I am naturally an aggressive person so when I was hit with Depression my aggressiveness tended to get the best of me.

One activity that always made me feel better is to take Loriann shopping for new clothes at the Pasadena Mall. I loved buying her clothes and how happy it made her and how beautiful she was in the new outfits. We had

bought some tights for her that had a tear in them from the start. So, we

went into the shop to return them and there was a man with a foreign

accent, and he refused to exchange them or return them for us. Well, the

mixture of my Depression and my Aggressiveness were a volatile mixture

and my aggressive nature kick in. I really started to have a heated verbal

confrontation with the man that escalated quickly. Loriann was doing

everything possible to settle me down, but it was too late I was so upset

and fuming and my feelings were only accentuated by my Depression. I

actually started to go over the counter after him. Security was called on me

and I was escorted out of the store. After things settled down emotionally

and I could see how upset that I had made Loriann, I realized that I was

completely out of control because of the Depression. I was embarrassed

and felt terrible for what I had put Loriann through. So, you need to be very

aware of our temper and your aggressiveness when you have Depression.

THIS MENTAL PAIN IS EXCRUCIATING

Loriann and I decided that we wanted to build a house. So, we just decided

to do it and make it happen. We found a beautiful acre in Farmington Utah

for an excellent price and somehow, we were able to come up with the money to buy it. It was so funny because we bought it from this funny older Dr. After we closed on the lot purchase, he stated " I forgot to tell you about the Volcanoes on the Property, it was way funny. " So, we had this absolutely beautiful piece of property to build on and we moved forward on designing a simple but amazing Ranch House with a Cedar Roof and Cedar Shakes. We had old doors that were all different styles and most of them were over 50 years old. It was one of the houses when people would walk in, they would say "Wow" which was fun for us. After I was finished with my regular job working on the Real Estate Development, I would come out to the house and work on it. I distinctly remember nailing the rows of 1.5-inch-thick Cedar Shakes and each row would take me about 30 minutes to complete. I remember one night everybody had gone and I was on the roof by myself nailing the shakes on the roof. I just remember only being able to think about the excruciating mental pain that I was having and that it was so intense in its nature, that I couldn't even focus on nailing the Shakes on to the roof. I remember throwing my hammer, satchel and shakes as far as I could throw them in despair. I was completely exacerbated by the intense emotional pain that I felt, it was literally encompassed every second of my thoughts, I just couldn't take it anymore.

Sometimes the pain gets so bad you just must get through it, and sometimes you must give in.

I CAN'T TALK, REMEMBER WORDS OR NAMES

For some unknown reason, your mind is in a general fog with Depression and your inability to remember names, and specific vocabulary words and being able to get your words out in a clear concise sentence is very frustrating. What is most embarrassing is when you see an item that you have known the name of for years and you can't remember what it is, or you have known someone for 30 years and you can't recall their name. Sometimes your sentence structure sounds like you have no education at all.

ALL THE DOCTORS I WENT TO

I went to at least 20 different doctors. They all thought that they had the solutions for my symptoms by providing some treatment or pill regiment, none of their pills, serums, liquids, treatments worked on me. I went to one doctor, where he had me take an initial dose of 100 pills to start the regiment, a 100 pills and another 50 pills per day which was just plain ridiculous. I went to another Doctor that gave me a weekly serum in a shot. He was 97 years old and I went to see him in his home office located in a mobile home park. One day I was getting my shot, and he said that he had better hurry up with my treatment because his son was coming over for lunch. Now he was very old at the age of 97 years old and I asked him how old his son was, and he stated " He is 78 years old" I found that absolutely amusing and comical that he had a 78-year-old son.

I went to countless Medical Doctors, Neurologists, Gastroenterologists, and General Practice Doctors. The final conclusion is that not one of those doctors had the answer. Why because the answer wasn't physical. It was mental, it was a Physiological Disorder called Depression. It was in my head just as some people earlier had told me, but I refused to listen because I thought people that had Depression were weak, oh how I wished I had pushed my pride aside would have been humble enough to hear what others were trying to tell me. So, don't waste thousands of dollars, tons of emotional energy, suffer huge disappointments and realize that you may really have Depression.

Depression is not sadness. Depression is not a bad day or a breakup or a failure in life. Depression doesn't feed off negativity, it creates it.

Depression isn't a result of negative thoughts. It can't be willed away by an hour of meditation or a good gym session.

Depression is the fear that engulfs me in a moment of fleeting happiness because I know it's fleeting. It's the insurmountable barrier between me and anything good because I won't let myself far enough to fall again. Depression is the snake in the bush watching me build myself up again piece by piece the way it watches its favorite prey.

Depression is not "fixable. Depression is often the bleak realization that I don't know why I'm sad. How do you a fix a problem without knowing why it's there in the first place?

Depression is the tsunami wave at 2 a.m. and 2 p.m. It is the weight of the world bearing down on me just when I thought I was free. Depression is my body caving in and vanishing into the black hole that has learned to hide behind my heart.

Depression is not disposable. It is not convenient. Depression cannot be controlled or tamed. It burns what it wants, takes what it wants and destroys what it wants.

Depression is unrelenting chaos in my mind, painting the world black. It is the tugging at my throat, at my heart, at my mind. Continuous tugging, pulling until all I want to do is fall.

Depression is not romantic or the plot of a tear-jerking movie. It is not beautiful or acceptable. Depression is not a commercialized product for people to pity. Depression is not "a part of a person" — it's what ruins a person

Depression is a party with your good old friends: guilt, anger, fear, and emptiness. It is a gala of my worst moments, my mistakes, and my regrets. A celebration of everything I am not and will never be.

Depression is wondering if I'll ever be better. It's the debilitating realization that no matter what, no matter where, no matter with whom or when: I may never be OK, perhaps for an hour, or a week or even a month — but not forever.

Depression is a mental illness. Depression is felt in spreading through my blood. It is the lead in my bones. It is the rocks in my heart. Depression engulfs me, drowns me, and suffocates me.

Depression is the deepest loneliness I will ever know in my life.

Depression is the only friend I let close enough to destroy me because if I

let anyone else close enough, my Depression will destroy that friendship

7

<u>YOU MUST HAVE COURAGE</u>

You cannot be weak and survive Depression. If you cannot come up with the courage to face this disease you will end up committing suicide. Your wife and children will have to deal with the emotional aftermath that occurs because of your lack of courage and selfishness.

You had better realize one thing, that facing Depression will be the hardest thing that you will do in your entire life, it will turn your life upside down and you will face emotional and physical trials that you didn't even could exist. Depression is an insidious disease, I consider it a very evil thing, and is so severe in its effect it is just purely overwhelming as a physical ailment.

So, when you come up against a monster, you can either slay the monster or have the monster devour you. At this point in this book, you need to literally sit back and decide.

DO I WANT TO LIVE AND BE WITH MY LOVED ONES OR DO I WANT TO DIE?

You need to make that decision now. I will influence you to live, because life is worth living, making it through this disease will be one of the hardest, but the most rewarding experiences that you will ever go forth. If you handle it right, you will be ten times the man you were before, and your character will shine. You must become a warrior, you must be tough, you must be strong, nothing can be allowed to defeat you, you will go forward and try your best to be fearless to slay this beast, conquer this disease and be victorious standing next to your loved ones. You must make a conscious decision to be tough, Depression is not for the weak and it will destroy you if you let it. You must decide now that this disease will not ruin my life, that I am strong, and I will face it head on and be victorious.

A man killing himself because of Depression should never happen because the people that live with him should be knowledgeable enough about the disease that they would take the appropriate actions at the correct times.

I coached basketball against an individual who called the police officers while his wife was away and told them he was going to kill himself with a gun, and they needed to be there before his wife came home. This is a life wasted, he never needed to do this, but because he or nor his family was equipped with the right tools or resources this tragedy occurred.

Another tragic event involved a multimillionaire Bishop of our sister ward He was released from being Bishop and that day he went home and got a shotgun, went in the shower, and committed suicide. This is a man that has a beautiful family, a successful entrepreneur, and now he is gone. If he had been equipped with the correct knowledge and resources this would not have happened.

As I hear about several different stories about men committing suicide because of Depression, I am very alarmed and concerned. My first response is that it is not necessary, and it should never get to that point.

Family members, siblings, and loved ones do not understand the real implications of Depression and just what the sufferers are up against. This is a daily battle that can really wear you out, but suicide should not be the only option that an individual should consider. I have been at zero hope and know what it feels like to have absolutely no hope and it is the worst feeling that you can feel. The good news is that there are answers to almost all questions and problems in life. But the key word here is awareness, being able to see that there is an answer to this problem and a light at the end of the tunnel is just temporarily out of order. What a tragedy for a man's world to be so discouraging and awful that suicide is the only option.

Even though they think that it is the answer they don't realize that they are loved by their babies, they do not want their father gone, they will miss him so badly, but the person is unable to see no other options and that is when suicide comes into play.

The key here is to make the man aware that options do exist, and he needs to believe that options exist in his mind.

One of the biggest problems there is that an individual is not willing to try to have hope and belief in options that may work. He must believe that he can be helped which involves mental toughness of which a lot of men just do not have, some men would rather be miserable and try to get others continual compassion.

The other problem is that others around them are not aware of what they are dealing with and the serious consequences of the disease. If they are not aware that they are unable to provide the options and make the man even believe. So, loved ones need to be educated and aware of what they are dealing with.

If you have Depression, you can't be weak, or the decks are stacked up against you from the start. Depression is much too hard of disease to be weak.

Men need to realize that when they come up against Depression, that they and they only are responsible to find an answer to their problems. It is not the wife or the family that is responsible. If this does not happen the likelihood of the man getting better is minimal at best.

There is an interesting paradox of why men commit suicide. Men are supposed to be masculine with Testosterone running thru their veins. They are supposed to be the aggressor, the hunter, the one in charge. They are trained not to show their emotions and not to cry. Yet when a man is faced with Depression he wants to reach out for help, he wants to show his emotions, he wants to cry, but he can't because of the stereotype that he falls under and how he needs to portray himself as tough and as the breadwinner and the protector.

8

MEDICATION

This is one of the most difficult chapters to write about because taking medication for Depression is so critical, but at the same time, it is such a hard thing to commit to.

Finding and taking the proper medication is the most important aspect of coping with the Depression. You are not going to get better from Depression by just visiting a talk therapist. You may feel better while you are there, but talk therapy is temporary.

Medication is the key. You may think I am not going to take pills to get me high. Let me make it very clear, these pills do not make you high. They simply raise the level of serotonin in your body to the level it should be at. I heard one commentator say, why they must get high by taking this medication. Medication does not make you high as some people make you believe. All they do is bring you up to hopefully the normal level of mental health. So, if someone tries to fill you with that garbage it is false.

Another statement that you hear is that I can do it with a stronger will. Will has nothing to do with it, you could have the strongest will of any human on earth and you will never take away the pain of your Depression.

You may hear other people say that you need to stop thinking so much about the way you feel. If they had Depression, they would be saying the same things. It is all consuming, unrelenting, and continual so it is very hard to not talk about it.

You may also hear that you just need to pray for God to help you to be strong. You will see that these are the things that people think will make a difference.

For Depression, the only thing that will make a major impact is medication. I don't want to take drugs, I will try something natural, how stupid are you, if God has provided the medical break thru and technology in medicine then why not use them. That is like saying, I know I could die from this infection, but I don't like to take drugs, so I am not going to take that polio vaccine you created. God created medicines to help mankind.

There are certain drugs that can speed up or catalyze another drug such that it will work better and faster.

The most common side effects will be headaches, nausea, and dizziness. These symptoms will go away in time, so you need to be patient.

I read an article about supplementing testosterone; I thought why I don't try that for my Depression. So, I had my testosterone tested and it was low. So, I had the Dr. Prescribe testosterone patches which have had excellent results. I have been taking it for 12 years. It only makes sense; males testosterone starts to decrease every year starting in your 20's. I figured this out twelve years ago and just recently the literature is coming out that supports using it as a treatment for Depression. Another great feature is that it slows the aging process and helps you keep your muscle tone.

I am not going to pull any punches, I am going to tell you exactly what Depression medication does to your body and to your emotions. First, you will never get better from Depression if you don't take medication for it. So, you might say to yourself, I have never been a person to take prescriptions and I don't believe in taking a prescription for anything. Well then you have absolutely no hope of getting better from Depression, you will most likely commit suicide and leave your family with the emotional shame that goes with that. The proper perspective is that you should feel fortunate that you live in an age where there are so many different medications to help you

with Depression.

The longer you wait to take the medication, the worse off you will be, the

sooner you take the medication, the better off you will be. So, you must

have the mindset that I have to take these prescriptions to fight my

Depression.

The second perspective that you need to have is that you may have to take

these for the rest of your life. What is your other choice, the other choice

simply put is you will commit suicide because you will not be able to handle

the emotional pain of Depression?

Taking medication is not easy, and if you have the idea that you are going

to be given a pill, take it and you will feel much better in the morning,

you're very mistaken. You need to understand that finding a medication

that will help you can be a very difficult task.

Finding the right medication for your body and mind is a long journey and it

doesn't happen overnight. A lot of people think that you are prescribed

medication and you feel better, that couldn't be further from the truth. You will try possibly over 10 different medications, so you must be committed to the medication journey

Medications are different for every person that takes them. The first rule of taking medication for men's Depression is this. If you take a medication and it makes you feel worse physically, it is the wrong medication and you need to stop taking it period. Now your psychiatrist will say that you need to give it time. Your symptoms will never get better with that medicine. So, stop that medicine and try another one.

Another thing about medicine is that if it is going to make a difference the second you take it. With medication that is going to be effective in the long run, I found you usually will be able to feel the emotional difference right away, possibly the same day or even the day after. This is always a good sign, and this is the right medication for you to stay on. Now some medications can take a week or so to work, but don't get sucked into the Dr's word saying that it takes time for it to work because that is false, they don't take that long to start working. These are words for you that come from experience.

A lot of psychiatrists will mix different medicines. This is ok and normal and does not be afraid if this is suggested by the Dr.

You do need to be careful on how many different medicines that you take, because they all have side effects and the less medicine that you can stay on the better. Remember that one day you will be coming off these medications possibly, so the less medication the better.

Anxiety is a huge part of the Depression. There will be times where you will feel like you are going to fall off a cliff, where you just want to die. I had anxiety so bad with my Depression that I literally couldn't physically stretch for over 15 years. Now it is rare that I will vouch for a medication on the market place but there is one medication that is the best medication on the market place. It works fast, has no side effects. It is called Buspar or Buspirone. It is so fantastic, you can be having severe anxiety and you take one and it will take your anxiety away.

There are things that you cannot take when you are taking medication. One of those things is you can't eat or drink Grapefruit Juice or grapefruits Another thing that you cannot take when you are taking medication are vitamins, minerals, or herbs or any supplements. These items neutralize your medications and take away the effectiveness of the medications don't take them

All medicines have side effects, this is the worst part of taking medications. The great thing is that they are making medications with less and fewer side effects

Medication is addictive. Your body will become addicted to these medications and when the time comes to get off them, which I hope happens to you, your body will have a physical addiction to the drugs. When I attempted to get off Zoloft, it was almost impossible because my physical body had a dependence on these drugs, even though my brain no longer needed them to achieve emotional equilibrium. So, don't believe for one second that they are not addictive physically because they are. Now you need to keep in mind that it is better that you take the drugs and have the benefits they offer to you and deal with the physical addictions symptoms you will face down the road, it is well worth it to have the drug to help you with the Depression.

Lastly, I would be doing you a disservice if I didn't tell you the real facts about what the medicine does. These medicines are built to alter your emotions, they are designed to suppress the painful emotions that come with Depression. Well, the bad news is that if they are suppressing the bad emotions that make you feel mental pain, that they naturally suppress other emotions that you may have. Another way to say it is that you cannot feel emotions as deeply when you are on most Depression Medication. You just won't be as emotionally sensitive to different situations, you most likely will not be able to cry as easy or be touched by emotionally touching situations. Your ability to really feel feelings deeply is impaired by the medication. But you do not have a choice here, if you don't take the medication, you have a good chance that the emotional pain will cause you to commit suicide, so the alternative of not being able to feel emotions as deeply as you normally is a good trade-off to stop the insatiable emotional pain caused by Depression .

9

PSYCHIATRISTS

A Psychiatrist is a Doctor that is specialized in prescribing the medication for Depression. One of the hardest things about dealing with Depression is finding a good Psychiatrist. Why is it hard? Because there just aren't that many great ones out there. This is the reality of the situation. Psychiatrists are usually not taking any new patients and are booked out about 2 to 3 months. You may get into a Psychiatrist that will take you, but that is not a good sign. It is kind of like a Restaurant, if you go there on Friday night and there is no wait time and the Restaurant is half full, you know that the service or food is most liking lacking in quality and substance. The same is with Psychiatrists, the good ones aren't taking new patients.

So, what do you do in this situation? The thing you don't do is go to a bad psychiatrist, a bad psychiatrist can take you down a very painful, useless, time-wasting path. A characteristic of a bad psychiatrist is that will not be very knowledgeable about different practices and medicines. As a sufferer of Depression, you must become a student of the disease. You must be up on all the latest innovative drugs and technologies, and you need to be able to present those to your psychiatrists. A bad psychiatrist is just worried about liability and is unwilling to listen to your ideas or different medicines and treatment and sticks with the safe medications that will cause him zero liability. These are the psychiatrist where you think to yourselves, why don't I just put up a sign and I could be a psychiatrist as I know as much as him. A bad sign of a bad psychiatrist is one that will get on his computer to look up the medicines that you are telling him about. When this happens, I would suggest you get up and run out of his office. This psychiatrist will do you no good and, on the way, out be sure to tell him not to bill you, you will bill him for doing his job.

So, what do you do? You must get a referral into a great psychiatrist, you must find someone who has had great results with a psychiatrist and tries relentlessly to get into that psychiatrist. Now here is the hard part, that psychiatrist may say no at first, but if you know that he is good, then you must be persistent, calling him twice per week asking for him to see you. Finding others that may be able to get you in to see him. Great psychiatrists are like gold, you must do whatever you have to get into them. DON'T GIVE UP, DON'T GIVE UP.

So, what do you do in the meantime until you get into a great psychiatrist? You must go to the General Doctor. This is a step that you need to take very delicately. You need to find a General Doctor that has had good results in prescribing Depression Medication. You don't just go to any General Doctor that has no idea what to prescribe, you must take control of your own health here and research the Dr. and find out if he has had success in the medicine he is prescribing, which includes interviewing the doctor and finding out what experience he has with different medications and treatments. You are paying the Doctor, so don't be shy in asking questions. If you he balks or is rude or won't answer the question you have, I suggest you walk out. This is too difficult of a process to deal with dumb or arrogant or condescending Drs. who aren't knowledgeable. Please just do it. Take control of your health. So, find a knowledgeable General Dr. till you can get into the Psychiatrist you desire to see. THE KEY HERE IS DON'T GIVE UP DON'T GIVE UP.

10

TALK THERAPY

The truth of the matter is that there are a lot of very weird strange therapist or Clinical Psychologists that you go to. For example, I went to a renowned Psychologist and he fell asleep on me. So, I just started talking about random things that didn't make sense while he was asleep and when he woke up, he said: " I agree". It was a disappointing experience. I can't tell you how many Psychologists who had a stereotypical look of pleated pants hiked up on their hips, unkempt beards, and jogging shoes. I went through a whole lot of different disappointing Therapists.

Let's discuss and clarify the role of the Therapist when it comes to your Depression. First, you will not get better with just doing talk therapy. That is the job of the medication, the medication is far above more important than the therapist. A good Psychiatrist is the ultimate key piece is getting your health back. The Psychologist is merely a piece of the puzzle.

Their purpose is not to get you better. Their role is to assist you in navigating the mental issues and problems that arise because of the Depression. The Depression will change the entire texture of your emotional life and your personal relationships, you will be dealing with issues and things that you would not otherwise deal with unless you had Depression. Show they are there to help you navigate around all the bumps and roadblocks.

Do not have your Psychiatrist be your Psychologist, these need to be separate members of your team, and the Psychiatrist needs to be the prescriber of medicine, while the Psychologist is the prescriber of information and solutions.

How do you find a good talk therapist? One very simple answer, trial, and error. You may go thru a dozen therapists until you find one that works for you. The key phrase is one that works for you. One who gives you strategies and answers that sit right with you, that makes sense, that work for you.

You need to have someone that you feel cares about you and is just not another a therapist charging by the hours. They need to care about you, and you need to feel that.

If your Therapist says or does something weird or creepy or doesn't make sense to you, get up and walk out this is too hard of a process to deal with lousy therapists.

You need to have a therapist that doesn't take the same approach to every single problem. A lot of therapists have cookie cutter methods that they use because they are too lazy to figure out how to do it the right way.

A bad therapist can damage your emotional state and set you back with your treatment. So be very careful of who you go to and be very aware of their treatment and if something doesn't feel right it probably isn't right and get up and walk out. They aren't working it, but your mental health is.

It is important that you know that you are being heard, that they are listening to you. If you know that they are not listening, then get up and walk out seriously, you need someone you are paying to put in the requisite amount of effort which includes listening to help you along your path to health.

11

YOU ARE THE ONLY ONE

Your life will continue a downward spiral until you come to the realization that you are in charge of your life, and you are in charge of our health.

When you have Depression, you tend to feel sorry for yourself. It is such an extreme and profound experience you can't help but feel sorry for yourself. The problem is that you want everyone else to feel sorry for you, but other people can in no way relate to what you are going thru or feel the emotional and physical upheaval that you are experiencing. You will find yourself telling anybody that will listen about the mental pain and physical symptoms that you are going through with Depression. The need for compassion almost acts as a drug for you, it makes you feel better, but it is always short-lived, and you are back having to deal with your Depression by yourself. A majority of people don't understand what you are going through and most of them will consider you to be mentally weak and will look down on you as a weak individual. That is a very harsh judgment to have, but it is true.

Do not outwardly search out people who will feel compassion for what you are going through, because they just don't care as they don't understand what you are going through. Why can't they understand, because what you are suffering from is the invisible monster of Depression, if you can see it, it must not be there. What am I leading to is this, YOU ARE THE ONLY PERSON THAT IS GOING TO GET YOU BETTER? If you are thinking that other people are going to get you better, you are mistaken, it must come from you, you must be the engine behind getting yourself better.

How do you go about doing this? I am going to give you the no. 1 key in this entire book of how you are going to start to get better. First, let me give you some perspective from my own life. When I first got Depression, I was so lost I didn't know what to do, so naturally, I was talking to a lot of different people about what was going on. The main person that I shared my mental physical symptoms with was my father; a surgeon of 45 years in Canada. He was a very kind hard-working man.

I remember telling him about it, and he said that I needed to stop thinking about it so much and stop talking about it so much and that there was nothing wrong with me. I was devastated by his words. He knew me, he knew that I had always been a hard-working ambitious genuine kid. I felt betrayed by my own fathers, and tears streamed down my face from the pain of those words.

The only person that really believed me was my wife Loriann, and how I loved her for believing in me. This is a good example of what you may face if you try to tell people what you are going thru.

Once you have decided to take responsibility for your own health it is essential that you do the following. Go outside to a place that is quiet and you are alone and state the following words. I TAKE FULL RESPONSIBILITY FOR MY OWN HEALTH AND PROCLAIM BOLDLY THAT I AM GOING TO GET PHYSICALLY AND MENTALLY BETTER AND THE GOD OF THIS UNIVERSE IS GOING TO HELP ME GO DOWN THIS PATH TO HEALING.

This is exactly what I did one day, and I testify that my healing started that day and most of all my mental mindset changed, I was now in charge of health and my life. It was the most important thing that I did in my entire process. You may think that this sounds stupid or it is not necessary to do this, once again I testify you that it works and if you were smart, I would let the universe start to work in your favor and daily, you verbally state aloud

those words written.

12

<u>ESCAPING THE MENTAL PAIN</u>

I am going to talk to you about the things that brought me relief from my Depression. What things helped me achieve relief may sound weird to you and may sound unnecessary to discuss, but this is something that needs to be discussed because what brings you relief will typically end up being very bothersome to the people around you.

For some reason watching TV brought me relief from the mental pain of Depression. I think the reason that it is it because the mental pain is in your thoughts 100% of the day, but when you watch tv it can completely consume all your thoughts, so you are thinking about what is going on the TV instead of your mental pain.

Another thing that brought me comfort was darkness. I loved the darkness when I had Depression. I used to put on my hoody and zip it up so that there wasn't any light and I would relax in the brown chair as is became known as.

Sleeping was a good way to get away from the mental pain because you were not in your conscious mind and therefore you didn't feel the mental pain.

Watching my kids play sports and coaching my kids in basketball relieved me of my mental pain because my focus was so strong on the game and coaching it and not on the mental pain. So, anything that requires you to have an interesting focus, I say interested because if you must focus on something you do not enjoy it won't work.

Let's talk about how your loved ones will learn to hate the things that bring you comfort. These things that help comfort you become your defaults of what to do if the pain gets unbearable. So, your family will see you zip your hood up, sit on the brown chair, watch tv, and sleep. They will learn to hate them because they see you doing them so often and they really don't understand that the only reason you are doing those things is that it is the only way to get away from the insatiable mental pain.

So, I think it is important to sit down with your spouse and your children if they are old enough and describe the insatiable mental pain to them and there are certain things that will give you comfort from the pain. That you do not do those things to be lazy or be a slouch, but those things give you comfort. They need to understand that. It got so bad with me, that the brown chair became very hated in our household, but little did they know that brown chair represented comfort from the pain of my Depression. So that really did hurt my feelings.

Sleeping really can bring a clinically depressed person comfort. There were times in my life when my two oldest kids were teenagers where I couldn't get out of the bed in the morning. It wasn't because I was lazy, I had proven to Loriann early in my life before I got a Depression that I wasn't lazy. But there are times where the pain is so excruciating that you can't get out of bed. Now if your spouse and your older children do not understand this and are not educated on this, they will turn on you, gang up on you and consider you not to be a fit father and parent. I know I went through this exact thing. So, you need to sit down and have a dialogue about the things that bring you comfort, and that you are going to have to use those things to get comfort when the mental pain from Depression is so bad.

13

<u>QUIT ASKING WHY ME</u>

I am going to state one of the most important things about Depression that I will tell you in this entire book. I was so discouraged about my Depression and I fell into one of the most serious traps that you can fall into when it comes to surviving Depression. Depression is lived in the conscious mind.

With Depression, the conscious and subconscious mind do not get along and are out to destroy each other. You can't live the problems that you are experiencing with Depression with your Subconscious Mind.

How does a Depressed person enter the subconscious mind? It is a very simple method. If you ask your subconscious questions using any of the adverbs such as What, Where, When, How and Why. You cannot ask yourself or your conscious mind questions using adverbs about your Depression. You cannot ask Why do I have Depression for example. Here is what happens when you ask Why do I have to have Depression. That question opens the door to the subconscious mind. Even though your conscious mind asked the questions, it opens the door to the subconscious mind and the subconscious mind will try to answer it. It will attempt to answer the question in the background of your brain as you are going about whatever you are doing, but the problem is the it will not be able to find an

answer to the question and it will search and search until you are so full of

anxiety and increased mental fatigue that you will be so much worse off

than before asking the questions.

So, the most important thing in coping with Depression is that you do not

get to ask yourself any questions that have the adverbs What, Where,

When, How and Why. There is no answer for this and all you will do is go

down the bottomless rabbit hole of the subconscious that has no bottom

and you will only complicate things extremely and you will feel worse

14

LET IT GO

Depression will cause you to wear down your spouse by continually talking about your problems. All your spouse wants is to give you an answer to your problems because she loves you, yet she is typically not equipped with the tools to give an answer.

Things are a bigger deal with Depression, and you will hang on to the littlest issue or problem. You will get upset at your partner if she does the slightest thing wrong and you will not let go.

When you have Depression in a family and you are the head of the household, this is a recipe for disaster unless you are equipped to handle it appropriately. First, you cannot let your Depression allow you to think that acting out or mistreating family members is an option, because that can wear on your family and eventually destroy your relationships with them. The most important thing to have is awareness.

Let me give you an example of how this occurs. If you have an argument with your spouse, usually you can talk and forgive and move on. With the Depression talking, you feel an intense desire to make your point and make it repeatedly again and again. This will eventually lead to you burning out your wife emotionally and she will not want to be around you because of it. My wife used a perfect term for it " Lawyering her". I feel guilty to this day for every putting through all the petty things that I held on too long.

So, this is what needs to happen. First, you need to tell your spouse that this is a real problem and that you may tend to hang on to things in an argument. Ask her if you ever do this to let you know that you are doing it and that it is very unhealthy and that she needs to point it out to you when you do it and let you know that you are hanging on to things. Try your hardest to recognize this and stop. The next step that you need to take is to apologize for your part of the argument and commit to trying harder and let it go

Let me give you a stern warning about this. This is something that I did so much, so often that I emotionally burnt my wife out. This is not what your wife is for, apply what I said, or you will be divorced. You will have an insatiable desire to hang on to unimportant items, but just stop because it will only cause you to lose the people you love the most

15

YOUR SPOUSE IS NOT YOUR THERAPIST

I loved my wife Loriann so much, she was a sweet compassionate vibrant young woman that I adored. I made a ton of mistakes when I started to suffer from Depression. She was my best friend, my confidante, my most trusted person that I knew. So, when I was during this nightmare, guess who got to hear about all the hard things that I was going thru; Loriann and that was a big mistake. It is difficult to know what the best way is to go about what to do when you don't even know that what you are suffering is Depression. But she had to pay the price of listening to my emotional garbage.

Your spouse is your spouse, they are not your therapist and you do not treat them like a therapist ever. They are not trained in mental health and they don't have professional answers to give you about what you are going thru. The most difficult part is that they loves you so much that she wants to provide you with answers, but they can't. So, it's not right that they should go thru the pressure of coming up for the answers to your problems You should not be divulging all your mental nightmares and concerns that you are feeling and expect her to be able to understand how she can help you.

The eventuality is if you treat them like your therapist that they will not be able to emotionally handle it and you will lose the love of your life.

You need to come to an understanding between the two of you will not talk about any of the emotional or physical symptoms that you are going through. They are not responsible for your care as a person with Depression. So as tempted as you may be to discuss with them what is going on with you physically and emotionally don't include them in on that conversation. This is a conversation that you are to have with your talk therapist and your psychiatrist.

What role does your spouse play regarding Depression? Let me explain how it finally worked in my marriage as to give you an idea of what is the best role for your spouse to have. My spouse and I decided that what we would do is when I was feeling bad whether it be physical or emotional that I would just tell her that I am not feeling very well. Most of the time she would feel empathetic towards me and ask me if I wanted to get in her neck. So, we would lay on the bed and I would rest under her chin on her neck and often I would have tears streaming down my face because of my

mental pain and the pure compassion she showed me. The role of your

spouse is to only show compassion towards you.

16

YOU MUST DO THESE THINGS

When you have Depression, it is almost universal that it is a hassle to do almost anything, it is the nature of the Disease, as a result, you will develop habits of laziness. I am going to tell you some things that you need to do on daily basis and even more than one time per day whether you want to or not. This is going to take some guts on your part to do these things, but please trust me and I will not lead you astray, I know how hard your journey is and I know what will make you feel better.

CARDIO WORKOUT

It is essential that you work out every other day doing cardio. It is also essential that you do Cardio that is hard enough that you are out of breath, that you feel endorphins from your work out. Being able to have endorphins released from your body is very advantageous to you and it is something that Depression cannot hamper, what do I mean by working out hard enough that endorphins are released? If you get your intensity level up to a certain intensity level, endorphin will be released, and they feel so good. So, you can be lazy and lack courage, or you can be fearless and move forward and work out for a minimum of 30 mins doing intense cardio every other day.

Now you will never want to work out when you have Depression, never, so you are going to have to really believe in the benefit of this for your Depression. If you have a spouse, you tell her that no matter what you make me go work out. Now I suggest that you listen to some rock and roll, some metal music or hip hop that will get you going and give you extra energy during cardio. Now if you are a runner, that is even better, as you can get even more endorphins released with running. It makes take you going 3 or more miles, but these naturally released chemicals are essential to you surviving this disease.

WEIGHT LIFTING

I don't know what it is about weight lifting, but when you do it consistently with heavyweights, it just makes you feel better. So, I would suggest that you do hard cardio or running or biking one day, then the next day you lift weights. It does not do your brain any good to lift light weights. To really feel good from lifting weights you must really push yourself to the edge and it must be done with heavy weight. The mental benefit comes when you are pushing yourself and you don't know if you are going to be able to do that last rep, something is released in your brain that makes you feel good. Now if you haven't been a weight lifter in the past, may I suggest that you start today, not tomorrow, start today. Read up, get a trainer, ask a friend to help you, but become an expert quick on weight lifting because it is one of the most beneficial things that you can do along this arduous trail of Depression. Please take me seriously, this is a critical thing for you to do.

DAILY MANTRAS

Now when I mention this you will say that you are not going to do this. I used to feel the same way about of positive affirmations or mantras until one day I tried it and it made a difference, it made a monumental difference, it literally put me on the correct path that I had not been on previously. There is something about stating aloud or verbalizing aloud that connects you with the Universe of Heavenly Father. It really works. I mentioned early in the book that when I was at Zero Hope, I did a Mantra aloud and it took me out of that awful and dark decrepit place of Zero Hope. Here are some Mantras that I say daily that has given me a foundation of faith, hope and believe in Heavenly Father.

- I AM THE ONLY PERSON THAT IS GOING TO GET ME BETTER WITH THE HELP OF HEAVENLY FATHER

- I AM GOING TO GET BETTER

- I KNOW THAT THE ATONEMENT OF JESUS CHRIST HAS THE POWER TO HEAL ALL THINGS

- I KNOW THAT HEAVENLY FATHER IS GUIDING ME IN ALL THINGS THROUGH THE POWER OF THE HOLY GHOST, BECAUSE of THE HOLY GHOST TELLETH ME ALL THINGS THAT I MUST DO.

I testify that these positive mantras build hope and faith for your recovery.

continued that streak that the bad things that happened consequentially would have never happened. Believe me go to the temple.

DON'T ISOLATE YOURSELF

With Depression, you are naturally going to have the tendency to isolate yourself. It is ok to not want to go places at times, but it not good to completely isolate yourself from others. It is the influence of other people that are usually going to help you down the path of Depression. It is people that are put in your path that are going to be instruments in God's hands to help you through your trials. So, go to church every week, go to church activities, occasionally go out with friends that will make you feel better.

17

<u>DREAMS NEVER DIE</u>

Despite suffering the ravaging effects of Depression, it is essential that you continue to keep your dreams alive. The problem is that it is so difficult to do. If you have had severe mental pain all day and into the night, all you can hope is for the pain to be gone in the morning. With Depression that is usually not the case and when you arise the mental pain continues on. So how are you able to keep your dreams, when the Depression's mental pain is slugging you in the stomach all the time. It is very simple, you have to do no matter how bad things get. How do you even remember your dreams with all the mental and physical symptoms that you are battling?

There is only one way to do it and that is about habit. You write down all of your dreams on a piece of paper. Every morning and every night you read your dreams and goals verbatim and you end with a verbal mantra that Heavenly Father is going to assist me in achieving these goals. You need to verbalize these goals allowed.

I think I may have just turned the corner on realizing my dreams, dreams are not contained, dreams have no boundaries or definition, dreams are free to roam in the imagination of our minds. Dreams are what keep us from going backward, dreams squash fear, lack of belief, and are the creator of thoughts and actions. It is dreams that are the catalyst for everything and are what makes things happen. One of the greatest gifts you can give to another person allows them to dream and to let them see and feel the greatness of your dreams and where it will take them. Dreams make you happy, replace despair, dreams are the fuel the natural reverberation of your own enthusiasm. How dull and small it is to not dream, to get stuck in the rut of just living when you could be lifted with the imaginations of your dreams. Dreams are bright colors, they are huge emotions, they are smiles, they are love, they are growth, they are the palpitations of the heart, the realization of the belief that you can do it, that your thoughts will become reality. Dream stealers are the plague that dissolves the apparitions of your dreams, who smash the beautiful colorful thoughts that scamper thru your mind during daydreams and sleep. Dream stealers are like a blanket of acid that destroys all the beauty that exists in front of your eyes. Negativity is not dreaming, the judgment does not color your dreams, it turns them into a dull black and white. Judgment chops the tall beautiful dream down one cut at a time, till the dreams are incinerated by the cold and cruel lack of belief that dream stealers have. Stretch out your dreams by lifting your hands in the air and smiling across the sky and screaming I have a dream and I love it, run away with the swiftness that comes from the energy of your dreams. Run to those who feel what you feel who lift you up higher than you are, those whose smiles are even greater than yours. Dreams are fresh, they are alive, they really exist and continue to grow as you allow your heart to feel the red-blooded emotion flow thru your heart as you smile your dreams on others. You can smell dreams, you can feel dreams, you can taste dreams and most of all you can live your dreams. Now living those dreams brings a sobering yet incredibly humbling and grateful feeling knowing that you made it, that faith has taken you over the finish line, tears flow as you fall to your knees, you did it, you look to the Sky you rise up and let your bright star stained eyes look again to the sky, with outstretched hand you beacon to the universe and out comes the cry of the dreams, I did it, I really did, I overcame people and judgments and illness, and lack of belief and rejection, loneliness', isolation but damn it I did it as the grateful tears roll down your smiling cheeks. It hits you, for so long you said the words no fear, they were no longer words, they were real, you crushed your fears and smashed thru that wall and just like your dreams told you, the fresh smell of your dreams were there, they were alive, they were real, even though you doubted they were real, they really were and oh it feels so good. So, go forth this day and imbue your dreams into others and help them to live again thru their dreams. Dreams are life, life is dreams and a man without a dream is dead. What is life without a dream, I'll tell you it is you just going thru the motion with the monotonous look of a pale cowardly individual who has let others, the world and the crushing circular thoughts of his mind control him such that his dreams are no more. Step forth, raise your fists, declare you are a dreamer, smash down those weaklings who declare normalcy, who declare their lack of belief, throw them and their useless propaganda by the wayside, step on their necks and grit your teeth and with the voice of a dreamer declare once again I will dream and I will dream big and I will dream repeatedly and again. I will seek happiness thru my dreams, I will give happiness with my dreams and the illumination and enthusiasm of my dreams will draw those that are good towards me a d my energy will ward off those who are unable to see because of the dark steed of normalcy that they ride, they can't see it and they never will. To dream is a gift that will grow and grow if you feed it with knowledge and good thoughts and productive actions. Life may try to crush your dream, but you can overpower and force out life if you have a boisterous belief that is unrelentingly and is constant with an enthusiastic intensity that can burn thru unfaith fewer situations. Flex your spirit, flex your soul, flex your emotions, and feel my brother I said feel the universal positivity that your faith in your dreams will bring. Dreams are like the constant ebb and flow of the ocean, you will always hear your dreams and they will always be a beautiful sound unless you are deafened by a tsunami of fear, lack of faith, and just dumb people whose visions are that of a blind man. Be humble, be sharp, be enthusiastic, look forward not back, be firm, not soft, be nice not mean, be bright not dull, do good not bad, shy from those who wither, and go to those who grow. Dreams I say are magic, they are the creator of thoughts which are the creators of action, which are the creators of happiness, which is the creators of a full filled life,

18

<u>RAISING CHILDREN WHILE SUFFERING FROM DEPRESSION</u>

Depression and raising children are a very sad topic for me to discuss. When you have Depression, it is literally impossible to give your children emotionally and physically everything you could give them if you didn't have the illness. So, you must have certain beliefs and expectations that will be different with you having this awful illness. First, let me tell you a little about the expectations that I had for myself. I absolutely raising my babies with my Loriann. If there is one thing that we both succeeded together at that was absolutely enjoying every moment raising our children and really being in the moment as we raised them. I would often time in the middle of an event or activity look in Loriann's eyes and say " Isn't this the greatest thing ever raising these babies there is nothing better and we are really getting the most out of this experience" for that I am grateful.

I remember that I was at one of my son's competitive basketball games. A father I was sitting next to me said " Well here we go again, another one of his games to endure" I said to him "What" He said that he got tired of coming to these games. I stared at him with a certain disdain. I said to him " There is nowhere that I would rather be that her right now watching my boy play basketball, I would rather be here than laying on the beaches of

Fiji". That is how I believed about being with my children.

 I knew that with Depression that playing with my kids, coaching them,

teaching them and just being with them was going to be very difficult. Why

because everything that I did physically or emotionally with them hurt me,

it felt like I had 1000 lbs. on my back as I was with them, but I didn't care

because I was not going to lose the opportunity to be with my kids. I felt

like I was partially paralyzed most of the time and it was so incredibly hard

for me to force myself to do things with my children. I knew that this is how

it was going to be and there was nothing that I could do about it, but I so

badly wanted to be a part of my children's lives that no matter how bad I

felt I was going to push thru it and be with them and I decided that I was

going to be pleasant and happy while I did it.

My son Jack would ask to go and practice tennis at nights. So, we would go

and hit balls for 2 straight hours, I loved it so much and cherish that

memory to this day, but Jack didn't realize how painful and arduous it was

for me.

I would take me Max when he was 3 years old and teach him to skate, we would go several times a week and when he got old enough, I taught him to play hockey. I absolutely loved every minute of the experience, but it emotionally hurt me so badly. He also doesn't know this, but I wouldn't trade helping him put on his hockey equipment and tying his skates as a five-year-old for anything. I loved it so much.

I would take my Jeffy and prepare him for Jr. High Tryouts. We would start a couple of months before tryouts and would go every night and shoot 500 shots, 100 free throws, dribbling drills, and hard physical drills where he would be so tired, but he always worked so hard. He doesn't know this, but that hurt me so badly emotionally, I can't describe the emotional pain, it is impossible to describe, but I wouldn't trade those workouts for anything, I loved them. I made the decision that I wasn't going to let the emotional and physical pain stop me from having these amazing experiences with my children.

I also made the decision up front that I was not going to let my Depression and the unhappiness it brought me to reflect at all with my children and my relationships with them. So, I decided that I would never get upset at them,

I would listen to them and talk to them about everything. Well happy to say that this is something that I did succeed at and I was able to not let the emotional effects of the Depression fade over into the relationships with my children.

You must decide that you are going to put your Depression in a box on the shelf and not let it out when it came to interacting and building a relationship with your children. So, when it comes to children and raising them with Depression, you must have guts, you must have courage, you must completely forget about yourself and your Depression because they can't understand our Depression when they are young. You must commit to being active with them and doing as much as a normal parent would do if they didn't have Depression. No matter how badly you hurt emotionally or physically you must do it, or you will look back and all you have is regrets. You really must suck it up and put all any symptoms aside. DON'T BLOW IT WITH YOUR KIDS. I coached 18 different competitive basketball seasons and coached my two boys in tennis for 5 years and I did it with excruciating emotional pain.

19

IT TAKES COURAGE TO WORK

Wow working a job as a responsible male is so hard when you have Depressions and yes it does take courage. I had just graduated from one of the top Business Schools in the Nation at the time. I also had graduated from USC's Entrepreneur Program which was currently ranked No. 1 in the USA and I had won Business Plan of the Year at the top program. So, I had tremendous courage while at college and suffering from Depression.

Since tuition was so expensive, I decided that I would get two degrees by paying the same price for one degree. So, just last year I take 24 credit hours per semester. It was very rewarding, but it was very tortuous. I had to prepare for exams 4 weeks in advance because I had six different classes that I was taking. Why do I tell you this, because one of the greatest attributes you are going to need to have a successful life despite the Depression is courage, sometimes you just have to gut it up?

I just remember that I had anxiety so badly while I was at college my body didn't have the ability to stretch, I couldn't yawn, and my body was like a tightened robe 24 hours per day. But I had things that I wanted to

accomplish so I just gutted it out.

My tuition at USC was around $15,000 dollars per semester in 1986. To

help pay for my tuition I sold my 1979 gorgeous navy-blue Corvette with T-

tops and bought a 1976 Ford Pinto. It was one pathetic car. I used to park

my car at a gas station next to USC, it was also where all the rich kids

parked their cars. There was one Rich Kid from Argentina that had a

Porsche Turbo Carrera, I always made sure that he was not around while I

parked my car and would run away from my car after I parked it so no one

would know it was mine.

When graduated I got a job Selling Commercial Real Estate as a

Commercial Real Estate Broker. I was on MacArthur Blvd in the summer in

my pinto. It started to overheat and before I knew it, the car started to

smoke and start on fire. I got out of my car with my new Double-Breasted

suite, white shirt, and new tasseled black shoes. I lifted the hood and the

car had a small fire going and a lot of smoke. So, I did the only thing

someone who wanted to stop further embarrassment would do I

abandoned the car and went home. I never even went back for it, to this day I don't know what happened to it. I paid $675 dollars for that car and we got 30k miles out it by putting metal shaving in the radiator to stop it from overheating.

At my graduation, Lee Iacocca from Chrysler gave the speech, and my dad was so excited about it, he immediately when over to the Jostens's rings and ordered me an amazing expensive graduation ring, that I am so proud of today. He said this calls for us to go and celebrate by going to the Sizzler Restaurant. He thought that Sizzler restaurant was so great, I didn't think so, but I thought it was so cute and adorable that he loved it so much and wanted me to go there to celebrate.

I started my career selling Commercial Real Estate as a Commercial Real Estate Broker. It was a very prestigious job and I was so excited to earn the big commission that came with the position. I remember the first day, and how difficult it was for me because I felt was incredible anxiety that was so bad. Once again it was like my body was like a tightening rope. Having your body like that is literally exhausting and trying to succeed in such a high-pressure environment while battling Depression was oh so difficult. The hardest thing that I remember was how I just couldn't come across to people I met with the way that I wanted to, I just couldn't emotionally connect with them because of my Depression. But I had an expectation for myself, and I was going to succeed despite the absolutely excruciating emotional pain and horrible physical symptoms. I was proud of myself that first year as I earned over 100k in commissions and was at the top of my class that I came out with. The point I want to make here is you can sit and not accomplish things with this disease, or you can put it up, have courage, face these horrific physical and mental pains, and just decide that you are going to succeed.

We moved to Utah, and I got a great job as a Project Manager of a 50 million dollars residential development project. My boss took me up to the ground and handed me 6 sets of plans and said " Build it" if you have any major questions or problems our door is open otherwise just figure it out. So, despite being so overwhelmed with mental and physical symptoms that at this point were so bad, I decided to gut it up and succeed at this job. I was in emotional and physical pain every hour of every day. I just remember thinking what it would be like to be normal and not to have to wake up and worry about suffering these symptoms. I would ask Loriann what it was like to be able to wake up and go about your day and not have to have this layer of problems that you must deal with on top of your job responsibilities. She would look at me funny, like what are you talking about, but with Depression, you not only have to worry about doing your job but must cope with all the symptoms that come with Depression. I did succeed at that job, and the project was a success, and the only reason it was is I decided that I was going to have the courage and not let the Depression defeat me.

20

<u>DEPRESSION STEALS YOUR PRECIOUS ASSETS</u>

THIS IS THE MOST IMPORTANT ADVICE THAT I HAVE IN THIS ENTIRE BOOK.

MAKE YOUR SPOUSE A PRIORITY AND SERVE HER AND HAVE A GOAL TO

MAKE HER LIFE BETTER BY SERVING HER EVERY SINGLE DAY OF YOUR LIFE.

Yes, Depression is a paralyzing disease, it literally is paralyzing, it makes it

hard to walk across the room. This does not play a factor when it comes to

your spouse. Your spouse is your Goddess, she is your piece of gold, she is

your most prized possession on the entire face of the earth, and there is

nothing, let me repeat there is nothing that will take this prized asset away

from you. I have some very sobering information, Depression can take your

spouse away from you. Why because it is so paralyzing to try to have to do

physical activities, chores, and jobs. It is the hardest thing about Depression

your desire to move and do physical activity is significantly diminished and

it is oh so hard.

You need to decide right now as you read this, that you WILL NOT LET

DEPRESSION AFFECT IN ANY WAY YOUR RELATIONSHIP WITH YOUR

SPOUSE DESPITE HOW DIFFICULT IT IS PHYSICALLY. THAT YOU COMMIT

THIS DAY TO DO ANY AND EVERYTHING TO MAKE HER LOVE HER LIFE AND LOVE YOU.

So, if you don't feel like vacuuming, you're already starting on the wrong foot. You need to make a list of all the things that will make her life easier that day and do them. For example, if her car needs the oil changed, change it shut up suck it up even if it hurts and change it. If the house needs vacuuming, suck it up and do it. If the laundry needs folding fold it and shut up. You are to be thinking of her first all the time when it comes to your spouse, you don't matter, and the way that you are feeling is irrelevant, as far as you are concerned you don't have Depression.

This issue is the very thing that caused me to lose the love of my life, I had the women that I dreamed about, I had a woman that brought me great joy, I had a woman that was a wonderful partner and mother. I didn't do what I am telling you to do now and I lost the person that means more to me than anything thing or person on earth. Oh, how I could rewind life and go back and realize how blessed I was to have my Loriann. It is very difficult for me to read this and tears run down my face and they won't stop, because I lost my Lori, and there isn't a second, a minute, an hour, a day, a month a year that I don't feel sorrow for my stupidity and my inability to realize that I was destroying a relationship with my Depression and its habits. I miss her every waking moment of my life, I loved Loriann and I still do.

It took being alone and really submitting to my trials to have heavenly father through the holy ghost reveal to me all the ways that I needed to change as a man. I am grateful for my Depression, I know that may hurt for you to hear, but I am, after a year of being separated, I decided that I was going to become the man that Loriann most likely wanted and who heavenly father wanted me to become. I humbled submitted to Father and asked him to make my weaknesses strong and to refine out all the bad. I am humbled to say that I feel confident before god about my righteousness and who I am as a man. The sad part is that Loriann is gone, I lost the person I love the most on the earth. She doesn't know the man I am, she doesn't know the improvements I have made in my character and beliefs. I don't even believe the same anymore as I did before all of this. I am a good improved loving man, but I am this man by myself, only me knows how I have changed and the most important person to me doesn't even know how I feel and how I have changed.

So, from this day forth, I exhort you with every fiber of my physical,

spiritual, and emotional being that Depression doesn't matter when it

comes to the most important person in your life, your spouse.

So not only the physical things you need to do for her, but there is the

emotional side of things. I guarantee that your Depression has drained your

spouse physically emotionally and spiritually. I guarantee that and don't

think for a minute that it hasn't. You need to make up for this with your

spouse. How do you do this? You listen to hear when her mouth opens you

shut yours and do not open it until she is completely done. If she needs to

vent, you shut your mouth and nod your head and you agree with

everything that she is saying, because she is right, and you have already

drained her with your Depression. You owe it to her. Listen to her stop

talking and listen to her. Ask her every day how she is doing and if there is

anything you can do to make her life better. Look in her eyes 5 times a day

and hold her tight and tell her that she is the most important person on the

earth to you. Write her love letters stating how you feel about her, leave

her notes in her purse in her car on the mirror telling her the great things

that you love about her. Open her door always, push her chair her always.

Pray with her every night and pour out your heart to heavenly father in a genuine fashion telling him in front of her how grateful you are for your

spouse. Never ever raise your voice to your spouse. It is wrong. Never call

her any names but a sweetheart.

Never argue with her, there is one thing that I have learned by losing my

Loriann, there is literally nothing work getting upset with especially with

the love of your life. Oh, how I could go back and shut my mouth and just

smile and listen to her and really heard what she was saying.

I implore you to do as I have said in the words above, don't make the worse

mistake I have ever made a put myself and my Depression before the

person that Heavenly Father told me to marry, I blame myself and I regret

every day of my life for my selfish actions.

All I can do know is get better as a man, but I have to do it myself and no

one knows but me, when if I hadn't been so selfish and would have had

someone tell me how to handle Depression and treating my spouse, I

would be able to be a good man with the Love of my Life Loriann.

I lost the love of my life, the person that I loved more than any person on

the face of the earth, the person that made me smile, she was sweet, she was good, and she was kind. I lost my spouse and it is completely my fault because I let the Depression win over her.

This is a poem that I wrote describing me trying to catch the love of my life; Loriann's eye across the room, but it's too late she won't look at me and all I am left with is the regrets of what I could have done differently. I hope you can feel the pain in my words as I describe how I am trying to get her to just look across the room at me as our son opens his mission call. The objective is to show you how serious of a disease you are dealing with and if you don't handle it properly you could be just like me and lose the best thing you ever had. Here it is

ACROSS THE ROOM

The fresh love it brings tart dreams that taste so sweet.

Together your love can break walls, divide seas, lift your souls overall.

You PDA, your giggles, your youthfulness, and your Elders gaze back with slight disdain,

Just let a slice of life fill your pallet, see if you don't choke away those fresh vibrant, but immature dreams.

Children together, soft sweet kisses, vibrant smiles filled with belief, constantly adorn your attire.

He is so great, isn't she the best, these thoughts will never dissipate.

Your eyes meet across the room, and that warm tingle is felt in your heart and the assured feeling that she's mine forever, and how lucky am I.

Like an innocent pup, she greets you at the door and wraps her legs around you, hello my love, yet only a few minutes you've been gone.

Her insatiable desire to love and nurture your children provides quiet confidence that you chose well.

Her anguish over minor pains felt by your babies creates a deep appreciation for your decision.

Although some may have angst with their choice, you can always return assured that you are ok with her.

Nothing will ever change that reassured look across the room by each other and the silent eyes that say I just love you.

As things age up, the proper care is replaced by impatient empty moments of oh, she'll be ok, well he can deal with that.

Like a thief in the night, that warm, confident, believable love becomes second hand to the upbringing of teenagers abounding.

You feel a bit lost, a bit took back, a sullen sadness starts to pervade your spirit that is unfamiliar and unkind.

Yet you trust the altar for what it was made for, eternal love and your faith abounds in the promises made.

Stark pronounced words abide more often and with discomfort.

You gaze across the room is replaced with an unconfident stressful look of disdain.

It's uncomfortable, and for the first time, doubt leads to the stonewalling of warmth and love.

Outside there is a help, but their voices are foreign and insincere, nightly you plead for the effort to reignite what was.

Amidst the hurried pace of the created life before you, you look across the room hoping and honestly praying to catch her eye.

But all you feel is the strident effort by her to not look back at you.

Your heart aches, you have faith, but suddenly it's not enough, nothing does suffice.

Stained pillow cases are the norm and the constant discomfort of heart pain is unceasing.

That look across the room is to no avail, the love, the eternal promise, the gaze that was love is no more.

Pain, heartache, a war of words, disbelief, fruitless faith, and love lost.

There is nothing that can suffice the loss and the love that's there but is lost.

Time passes and passes again, your heart is to heal, but not so, you still have faith in that look across the room and the magic it held.

Accomplishments move forward, proudness prevails, calls to serve distant lands are had by yours so proud.

As the call is proudly proclaimed and read by the son of you both, your mind softens and for an oh, so moment time suspends.

The two of you sit and together are reading about future promises of your son's serving missions.

The warmth of the thought is profound, but slight because as the words North Carolina are heralded all you really want is for the gleam of your tears and hers to meet across the room.

The words silently unspoken but o so deeply felt, our boy he did it, he will serve the Lord

Once last time you look for your eyes to meet across the room

It's too late the look it isn't there and regret is the only thing to look upon.

By Robert Taylor

21

<u>SETTING PROPER EXPECTATIONS</u>

It is important that you have a family meeting to discuss in detail the specifics of the Depression, having the expectations and any questions that the family and children may have. You need to reassure them first off that you are going to be ok and that Dad isn't going anywhere, and that Mom and Dad love each other, and they are going to stay married. Then you need to lay out in a very simplistic format the specifics of Depression but in a format and a fashion that your children can understand in a loving way. You in no way want to scare the children or make them think that their Dad is going anywhere such as dying.

These are a hard expectation that the children need to hear such as the following. There are times where Dad will not be able to go and play with you. There will be times when Dad will have to stay in bed some mornings. There are times when Dad will not be able to go places with the rest of the family. There will be times when Dad is very quiet, and that does not mean that he is mad at you, it just is that he isn't feeling as good as he usually does. Sometimes you will see Dad cry, and that is ok. There are times where Mom will be holding Dad in her arms, and that is ok as Mom is just showing that she loves Dad. There are many things that you can talk about, but it is important that the children understand that this is a real problem, and just because you can't see it that it is real, and Dad does suffer from it.

Then you need to answer their questions in a loving way and reassure them that everything is ok, and things are going to be ok and that as a family we can stay stronger and we can love our dad and support him and as a family, we will become stronger as a result it. It is important that this meeting starts with a prayer and end with a prayer. This needs to be a teaching opportunity for all involved and if possible, you really need to have the spirit of the holy ghost there. The way that you do this is by inviting the Holy Ghost at the start of the meeting by inviting it in thru the prayer. I would suggest that you end the meeting with a fun activity and a fun treat, so the whole experience is a good one.

The main thing that needs to be the focus and come across to the children, is that this is a trial, and when then are trials when can get thru them and we can get thru them together as a family and the way that we get thru these trials is we stick together in faith as a family and mostly we love each other through these trials.

I can promise you that if you will do this, it will set the stage your family to become stronger through this trial. It's all about expectations and realizing that with family there is power, there is power in unity, their power in faith and that the gospel of Jesus Christ is the answer to all problems in life including physical problems such as Depression.

22

THE HOLY GHOST AND DEPRESSION

The Holy Ghost interacts with individuals with Depression differently than it does with people that do not have Depression. That does not mean that you are any less of a person, or that you are lacking spiritual strength, those things just are not true.

People in the Church or your loved ones that are members of the church will say absolutely say things to you that are completely stupid. You are going to hear things like " Just pray harder and you will feel better". This is false, prayer will not make you feel better. They will also say " Just read the scriptures and you will feel better" This is another false statement. " Have you tried fasting" What a ridiculous thing to say. I feel strongly that you will get better" These are all false statements and very damaging statements for you to hear. You may have these words even come from an uneducated Bishop which is very difficult to overcome.

God does not love you less because you have Depression if anything his heart is hurting more for you and he feels godly love for you.

You need to understand that all these statements that people will make to you are made from an uneducated basis, and most likely they are not trying to hurt or offending you, they think that they are helping you. You will have those who think that it is their duty to tell you those things and those people are usually condescending of how they deliver their opinions to you.

There are some people who you may love that will insist on giving you their opinion on this over and over. This is when boundaries need to come into place with those very aggressive opinionated people, for your survival you can't be around those people as they are hurting your wellbeing.

Do you feel the physical sensations of the Holy Ghost when you have Depression? First, let me explain what I mean by the physical sensations of the spirit , it feels like what I call it " QUADRAPLEGIC GOOD PIMPLES" it was a literal physical manifestation of the holy ghost. This is one of the saddest parts of Depression and it brings me to tears as I read this is the reality of Depression. YOU MOST LIKELY WILL NOT FEEL THE PHYSICAL MANIFESTATIONS OF THE SPIRIT WITH DEPRESSION. It may be different for you and I really pray that it is but with me I never felt those warm physical feelings or physical sensations that came with feeling the spirit. This is probably one of the hardest things that I had to come to terms with Depression. This is a very tough reality to face for you and I feel empathy for you and feel complete sadness that this is the truth.

Now does the Holy Ghost still can guide you in all things. It is stated in the scriptures that the Holy Ghost will show you all things that you must do. Does the Holy Ghost still guide you in your life with Depression, absolutely? It will let you know when you are making the right decisions and he will give you a stupor of thought if the decision you are making is the wrong one. So that is really reassuring that despite not feeling the physical manifestations of the spirit, you still will be guided on a continual basis by the Holy Ghost.

Let me tell you how the Holy Ghost will manifest itself with Depression. The only way that I know how to describe what I am trying to explain to you is through telling my experience. I was blessed with a kind, compassionate, empathetic spouse Loriann, who just wanted me to feel ok and be happy. If you are fortunate enough to have a spouse by your side that loves you as I did in Loriann, you are very blessed. When my Depression would get unbearable and I knew that I was on the verge of tears. I would ask Loriann if I could get in her neck as I called it. She never refused me once, she would lovingly take me to our bedroom, and we would lay on our comfortable California King bed and she would put me in her neck. I would often weep, and I am now as I write this, for her to never ever refuse me the chance to get in the warm comfort of her neck is just so unconditionally loving to me. I am so grateful to have had that. No word was said, we just held each other in a warm loving way and after a while, I would say I feel better, she would give me an embrace telling me things will be ok and that she loved me. What does this have to do with the Holy Ghost? I could feel the pure love of Christ throughout my whole being and spirit as loriann held me and I nuzzled in her neck. The holy ghost manifested itself through the pure love of Christ that Loriann showed me and I did indeed feel physical, mental, and spiritual comfort from the holy ghost through Loriann's Love.

23

SANCTIFY YOURSELF

This is going to be a very hard chapter for a lot of you to read. But I am writing about it because it was something that helped me a lot. When Loriann first separated from me, I was very bitter. I had decided that when I got married, I was going to completely focus on my family and my spouse. So that is what I did, so when Loriann wanted to separate from me I was very bitter and felt that she had abandoned me in the middle of my Depression. I was rude, angry, mean, hateful the first year or two and it just didn't do me any good. I also started to question things in the gospel, such as is it important to be obedient to the commandments and believed that it only mattered if you loved people. I was having a hard time understanding how when I gave 100% percent to my family and my spouse, then why is she wanting to separate. Well after 3 years Loriann decided to file for divorce. I was completely devastated. The only one on my side was Jeffrey my youngest who was 12 at the time. I remember feeling so sad for Jeffy, there were times that he would be with me and he would put his head down and weep uncontrollably for a few minutes. When Loriann filed for divorced he called up his 2 oldest siblings Max and Bridget and crying stated " Thanks for taking my dad away" There just is no power in separation and divorce, all the power of the gospel and the Temple just seem to fade away in insignificance.

Well, about 3 years in, I decided that I was just going to focus on getting better as a man and literally take an inventory of all my weaknesses and make them strengths, so I set out on that Journey while suffering severally from Depression.

The reason that I am telling you this, is that I was not a dedicated disciple of Jesus Christ, I was just Luke Warm, the scriptures really had no meaning to me, the atonement had no power for me, I wasn't really trying to live my life by the holy ghost and to put it mildly I count have been living the commandments a whole lot better. Well as time progresses, I decided that I was going to read the scriptures every single day without fail and I was going to pray twice a day. I continually prayed to Heavenly Father to help me to live the commandments must better. I made a resolve to live the commandments 100% percent and to repent 100% of a prior sin and for once to become clean and let the blood of our savior atone for my sins.

Well, once I decided to do that my whole life changed. I had struggled to find the peace that they talk about in the scriptures, the scripture " All ye that labor and are heavenly laden come unto Christ and I will make your yoke strong. I read about how to apply the Savior's atonement to feel peace and to be healed by the atonement. I really tried to apply the principle of first believing and having faith, then fixing anything that was wrong through repentance and then the Lord will take over.

There I law that states that the Redemptive Power of the Jesus Christ's Atonement is more available the more that you repent and sanctify yourself. I can testify to you the power of sanctification and that it works. I feel the peace from Heavenly Father now in abundance. I feel the spirit as much now as I did on my mission. I have always wanted to feel the spirit of the holy ghost like I felt it on my mission. Mine now pray with meaning and intent and focus, and when I pray, I feel as if I am communicating finally with Heavenly Father and not talking to myself. I cry tears from feeling the spirit all the time. I feel the spirit during the day a lot and I find myself saying " Thank You Heavenly Father" all the time.

If you are a Luke warm disciple, if the scriptures don't really have much meaning, if you are simply just rehearsing words in your prayers, if you are not feeling any peace from Heavenly Father, if you wouldn't feel confident standing at the Bar of God currently then may I challenge you because it nothing feels better than feelings clean. May I also challenge you because your journey down this path of Depression will be so much easier, so much easier. Please don't brush this off as religious speech, or that I am preaching to you. I have lived this, I have experienced the power of repentance during my Depression, and I testify that I would never have been healed from my Depression without repentance.

24

ATONEMENT: FOUNDATION FOR YOUR RECOVERY

The Atonement of Jesus Christ is essential to you coping with Depression, and to finally asking Heavenly Father to heal you of this disease. If at this point of this book you have not come to believe this, then you might as well stop reading as you have missed the whole point. The Atonement of Jesus Christ is powerful redemptive characteristics to it. So, I thought the best way at this point for you to understand that it to try to feel it. They say I can't remember what they said but I can remember what I felt. With that said please read this story about atonement that I wrote called

JOEYS DREAM

My father had just passed away, and I was just a young boy. I didn't understand why he had to die and if I would ever see him again. I had been told I would, but really wasn't sure. As I watched the grief of my mother thru the days, it weighed heavy on my heart. Will I see my dad again, or is that just a story?

As I went to sleep that night, I found myself thinking about my dad and the fun we had together. I would miss him and wondered if I would ever see him again. I started to fade and soon it was all I could do to keep my eyes open. I started to think about Jesus and how I had been taught that because of him we will be able to live again with my dad. I thought of how Jesus was nailed on the cross and how he bled from every pore. My thoughts turned back again to my dad. I could picture him perfectly. I could hear his kind friendly voice say to me Well Hello Joey, how are you. Whenever he saw me, he would always say hello. That just made me feel better, and when I thought of that it made me sad to think that there was a possibility that I would never see him again. My dad was so fun, he always liked to laugh and joke and have fun. Sometimes he was just downright weird, but he was my dad and I was going to miss him. I knew he loved me and being a boy of just 11 years life seemed it would be difficult to not have him around.

Finally, I succumbed to sleep. Suddenly I found myself lying down in the grass looking at the stars. Beside me lay my little brother Jessie. I nudged him and asked him where we were. He commented that he did not know. Is this a dream, I didn't know, I asked Jessie and he said I think this is real, but I soon knew that I was the most real dream I had ever had. I got up from the grass, pulled Jessie up and said come on let's go. The stars were so bright, and everything seems so vivid, the smells, the colors, and the sounds. We continued to walk thru the grass and approached a clump of trees. Thru the glimmering light, we could see the faint silhouette of an individual kneeling down beside a rock. We slowly approached the trees and hunched down to see what he was doing. What we saw was the anguish of a tormented man, never had I seen the grimacing on a man's face such as this, it was if he was literally fighting for his life. I could see the tears well up and flow down his cheeks. Jessie nudged me as said, that is Jesus, I took a second look and it was Jesus. We slowly walked around the trees and approached Jesus by the rock. We realize that he didn't notice us, and we realized that he couldn't see us, but we could see him. I was humbled and dropped to my knees. As I looked upon Jesus, I felt such incredible sadness and compassion at the same time. His tears continued to flow, as we heard him say father let this cup passed from me. I felt tears coming down my cheek and looked over at Jessie and he was also crying. We were watching the savior of the world in the garden of Gethsemane. The spirit was so strong. It looked as if he was in physical pain and his agony was so real. I approached him and put my arm around him and told him it was going to be all right. That is what my dad used to say and do to me and it always made me feel better. I also thanked him for doing this for me and

Jessie. He didn't respond, but all I felt was that the weight of the entire world was on his shoulders. I noticed red blotches on his garment, and it was true, Jesus had been bleeding from his pores from the pain. Immense gratitude flowed thru my body, he was doing this for me, I had always been told that, but really didn't know what it was like until now. I felt so bad for Jesus; I loved him and wanted to help him but knew there was nothing I could do. He was slumped on the rock from pure exhaustion. I felt helpless, never had I felt so much love for another person. And somehow, I knew that he loved me even more. We heard someone coming down the path and hid in the grass. They were coming to take Jesus away. As they left, we followed them from a distance.

 Next Jessie and I found we in a Courtyard with a whole bunch of angry people gathered together. Upon the balcony was a man in a fancy robe and Jesus was standing next to him. I heard him say this man is innocent. Suddenly the man next to me yelled crucify him, crucify him, I pushed at him and yelled stop, stop that is Jesus he only loved you, he never did anything to you, yet the man had no reaction and I realized he didn't know I was there. The entire group started to chant crucify him, crucify him. These people hated Jesus and you could feel a strong feeling of hate from the entire crowd. I couldn't believe that they hated Jesus and he didn't do anything wrong. My heart was hurting for him, yet there was nothing I could do. They were going to crucify him.

We next found ourselves in another courtyard with those same angry people. There were soldiers there and they had all these strange looking pieces of leather with metal objects tied to them. I thought, are they going to use those on Jesus. I couldn't imagine being strapped with those, even one time. A soldier approached Jesus and cut his garment, then literally ripped it off him. All that was left was a small piece of clothing barely covering his lower half. The soldier then took his hand and pressed the ring of thorns into Jesus's head. Why was he hurting him, and why wasn't Jesus fighting them at all, it was if he knew that he had to do this. I turned my head away because it was so hard to see someone is treated like that. The guard then tied his hand to a post and kicked him to the ground. The other guard yelled, now you will get what you deserve. I looked up at the guard and he had one of those awful whips in his hands and approached Jesus. He started to hit him with the whip repeatedly, every time Jesus would wince in pain. I started to cry and wanted them to stop, but they wouldn't, they seemed to be enjoying it. Finally, I ran and clutched the Roman guard around the waist yelling stop, stop he hasn't done anything to you, but to my displeasure, he didn't even recognize my presence and he didn't know I was there. Why are they doing this I yelled at Jessie, he is innocent and hasn't done anything wrong? They continued to whip him, and the blood from the wounds pooled at his feet. I put my hands in my face and could still hear the grimacing of Jesus and that awful sound of that whip. There was nothing I could do about it. I felt overwhelming love for Jesus and compassion I never knew I could feel.

I lifted my head up and it was silent. We were in a long corridor lying on the cobblestone. Jessie was next to me. We could hear the roar of an angry crowd at the end of the corridor. We ran to see what it was, and it was Jesus stumbling along the path with a great big cross on his shoulders. He was ragged and his face was stained with blood from the thorns on his head. I said to Jessie, we need to help him. Jessie asked how we would do that. I looked around and saw a fountain with water. Beside it was a discarded wooden cup. I grabbed the cup and filled it up and hurried down the corridor, Jesus was steps away from us. Suddenly he fell and the cross landed on top of him. He lifted his head up and he was looking directly at Jessie and me. This time he knew we were there. We quickly propped him up and Jessie gave him a sip of water. He replied faintly simply thank you.

The guards hit the cup out of my hand and pushed his face into the

cobblestone. Jesus arose slowly and stumbled down the way. I asked Jessie

what we should do. Jessie said why we don't carry it for him, the cross. We

fell back behind the crowd and waited for the chance to do so. Jesus

stumbled again, and we yelled to the Soldiers let us carry the cross for him.

I couldn't believe what happened next, the soldier whipped me and told me

to get out of the way boy. We were determined to help Jesus, so we

worked our way to the front of the crowd and both of us hoisted the cross

on our backs as Jesus fell to the ground. We looked back and saw

something I will never forget. Jesus looked at us as to say thank you for

helping me. It was painfully sweet; we were determined to carry it the

whole way for him.

As we traversed up the Cobblestone path, I knew it was Golgotha and was

aware of what was going to happen. I didn't want it to happen and didn't

know if I could watch it. We got to Golgotha and the soldiers pushed Jessie

and I down and the cross landed right on top of us. It really should have

hurt but I felt nothing as I looked back at the grimacing face of Jesus.

Everything seemed to go in slow motion from this point. I saw them lay the cross on the ground. They pushed Jesus towards it, and then literally dropped him on the hardwood of the cross. Again, we rushed the soldiers and told them to stop, but they threw us off like we were rag dolls. I couldn't really believe that they were driving spikes into his hands; I started to cry uncontrollably and didn't know how to help him. I fell to the ground with my hands on my face and yelled please stop, you are crucifying my brother and I love him. They nailed him to the cross and started to raise it up. They got it half way up, but it fell with Jesus underneath it. They really were going to crucify the savior of the world. The pain I felt for Jesus in my heart and compassion was indescribable. As we watched I became fixated on Jesus's face and I knew that he knew what he had to do. I knew he was doing it for Jessie and me and I was so grateful. When the soldiers left, I approached Jesus, I knelt and put my hand gently on his foot. Sobbing and hardly being able to get the words out, I told him I was so sorry and that I loved him, he looked at me, said nothing, but I knew he heard me. It was all I could do. There was nothing more I could do; he had to do it himself. I heard him faintly say "Father why has though forsaken me", the sadness wailed up inside of me, he was hurting so bad.

I could hear the tears of a woman behind me. I didn't know who it was, but it appeared to be his mother. I kneeled beside her and put my arm around her and told her how sorry I was. I looked up and heard Jesus say "Forgive them for they know not what they do" I couldn't believe he could still say those words.

I faintly heard someone calling my name and didn't know who it was. I felt the soft touch of a hand on my cheek. She said Joey time to wake up. I sat up on the bed, and tears filled my eyes. My mom said what is wrong; I said nothing is wrong; everything is going to be okay Mom. We will see Dad again and we will all live together again. I reached out and wrapped my arms around her and said we will mom we will see dad again I know.

25

<u>MIRACLES DO HAPPEN</u>

I have been anguishing from Depression for over 30 years. It has been a very distressing, formidable, and an enormously arduous experience that has sculpted me into who I am today. 4 weeks ago, I had about of Depression that was dark as dark, malicious, and totally consuming in its effect. It was an exceptionally depraved experience and I am challenged to put into words the anguish that I felt.

I was seeking for the Nth time a resolution to my insatiable pain from Depression that I was experiencing. Customarily I view some youtube videos before I retire to bed. The YouTube Video Scroll had a video about Depression. I had listened to it sundry times and it so often seemed to be just words and had no real meaning or wasn't of great import. For some reason, I decided to heed the words of the talk and undertook to feel every word with the assistance of the spirit. Every word distilled thoroughly upon my soul and I heard and felt words that I was not cognizant of before. In tears, the video deliberated that there are times when the bitter cup is there and the only thing that you can resolve is to drink the bitter cup, so drink it and do not shrink. It stated that Heavenly Father is a god of

miracles and you can have a miracle in having your mind healed. I retired to

my bedside and I knelt down and I prayed to Heavenly Father about the

insatiable mental pain that I was nursing and how I felt about bearing this

burden and drinking the bitter cup of Depression for over 30 years. It was

truly an earnest supplication that I felt with every fiber of my spiritual

being. This time I truly communicated with my Father. I let Father know

that I was hurting exceedingly and that I had been hurting for oh so long

and can he please succor me. I prayed with faith, real faith, trusting that I

could have a miracle. Heavenly father, I want my Depression to be healed. I

had prayed so many different times for the same thing but so many times

only arose to have to drink the bitter cup again. It is very humbling for me

and tears stream down my face when I feel the gratitude to Heavenly

Father for the miracle he indeed did grant.

Heavenly father let the bitter cup pass and granted me a miracle after over

30 years. I am healed from my Depression, I no longer feel the angst and

mental pain that Depression constantly serves up. I am feeling emotions as

true emotions, I am feeling emotions as they are supposed to be felt. I feel joy as joy, anger as anger, sadness as sadness, love as love. I describe it currently as <u>MY SOUL IS STIRRING</u>.

 I have not had a great day ever in the last 35 years, never. Even if boundless things were happening, there was forever the mental pain in the background and if I wasn't having mental pain I was cognizant that it was right around the corner ready to punch me out. I no longer have to face the inevitable daily mental pains of Depression.

I have come to trust that all emotions are separate and distinct feeling that are sent from Heavenly Father thru Jesus Christ. These emotions are intended to be felt in their purest form, but the trials of life and the physical barriers that our bodies encounter cause us to not be able to feel these emotions in their truest form. When you feel joy in its purest form it feels like joy, but it is not a nominal feeling, it is not a slight feeling, the true feeling of joy is deep and intense and is so amazing that when you feel if you just feel as if you will burst. When you feel sadness in its purest form, it doesn't manifest itself negatively, the true form of sadness is propped up by the pure love that father lets you feel in your heart and it actually is a peaceful sadness. When you feel the excitement you feel it to your fullest, it consumes your body physically and you just want to scream because you feel so enthusiastic about what you are feeling. The greatest things about pure emotion are that you can be feeling insatiable excitement and enthusiasm and five minutes you can be feeling the pure love from a different experience and have tears flowing down your face and it isn't manic in nature, its real.

Pure emotion is the essence of life. I have had the negative filter of Depression my entire life and have been unable to feel pure emotion, but people that have not had Depression have had the opportunity to feel pure emotion, but they really don't and there is a reason why. In order to feel pure emotion, you have to have a foundation, and that foundation has to be the pure love of Christ in your heart. Having the constant desire to have a pure heart and the desire to do every word and deed from a position of love.

After my wife decided she didn't want to be married after 32 years of marriage and 5 kids, I was mad and rebellious the first two years, but then I decided that I was going to submit to god and the refinement that came from the pain of my travail. I intently prayed to Heavenly Father to refine my heart, to root out any evil thoughts, to remove any guile, stop me from holding grudges, gossiping and judging. I prayed incessantly to have the desire to love all people unconditionally. So when this miracle of health started to take place, I had already established the foundation of love in my heart, as a result, the pure emotions were able to manifest themselves. I speak as a humble submissive student and not as a teacher.

Along with the purity of emotions comes the emotions that need to be curbed or refined. The emotions of anger, fear, and impatience will rear their ugly heads in a profound way. I found myself getting set off by things that people said or did to me. I found my self-losing my temper and felt that I was disappointing Heavenly Father after he has allowed me to have these pure emotions. I have an obligation to control and curb those emotions if I want to have the blessing of feeling pure emotions.

These emotions are so strong and can cause you to be overbearing. I mean I can get myself revved up very easy and take myself to a high emotional state very quickly. So I am learning to not let my energy and enthusiasm be too overbearing.

I am so grateful to feel deeply, and am so grateful and humbled to be able to feel piercingly deep this day. I have been driving up the Canyon, listening and getting lost in the music I enjoy. Once I get to the top I put on Christ-centered music, and it is as if the heavens open up to me and I am able to really feel the spirit of the holy ghost. I haven't felt this spirt like this since my mission, As I listen to this music, I sit and tears stream down my face and they are tears of the spirit and tears of joy, and it feels so incredible. I am feeling thoughts as pure as if they came right from God and am able to interpret those thoughts and put them into pure action.